MW01672154

Plant-Based Meal Prep Cookbook For Beginners 2020

Easy, Simple and Mouthwatering Meal Prep Meals for Healthy Plant-Based Eating (28 Days Meal Plan Included)

By Jimmy Shallal

Legal & Disclaimer

The information contained in this book and its contents is not designed to replace or take the place of any form of medical or professional advice; and is not meant to replace the need for independent medical, financial, legal or other professional advice or services, as may be required. The content and information in this book has been provided for educational and entertainment purposes only.

The content and information contained in this book has been compiled from sources deemed reliable, and it is accurate to the best of the Author's knowledge, information and belief. However, the Author cannot guarantee its accuracy and validity and cannot be held liable for any errors and/or omissions. Further, changes are periodically made to this book as and when needed. Where appropriate and/or necessary, you must consult a professional (including but not limited to your doctor, attorney, financial advisor or such other professional advisor) before using any of the suggested remedies, techniques, or information in this book.

Table of Content

Introduction

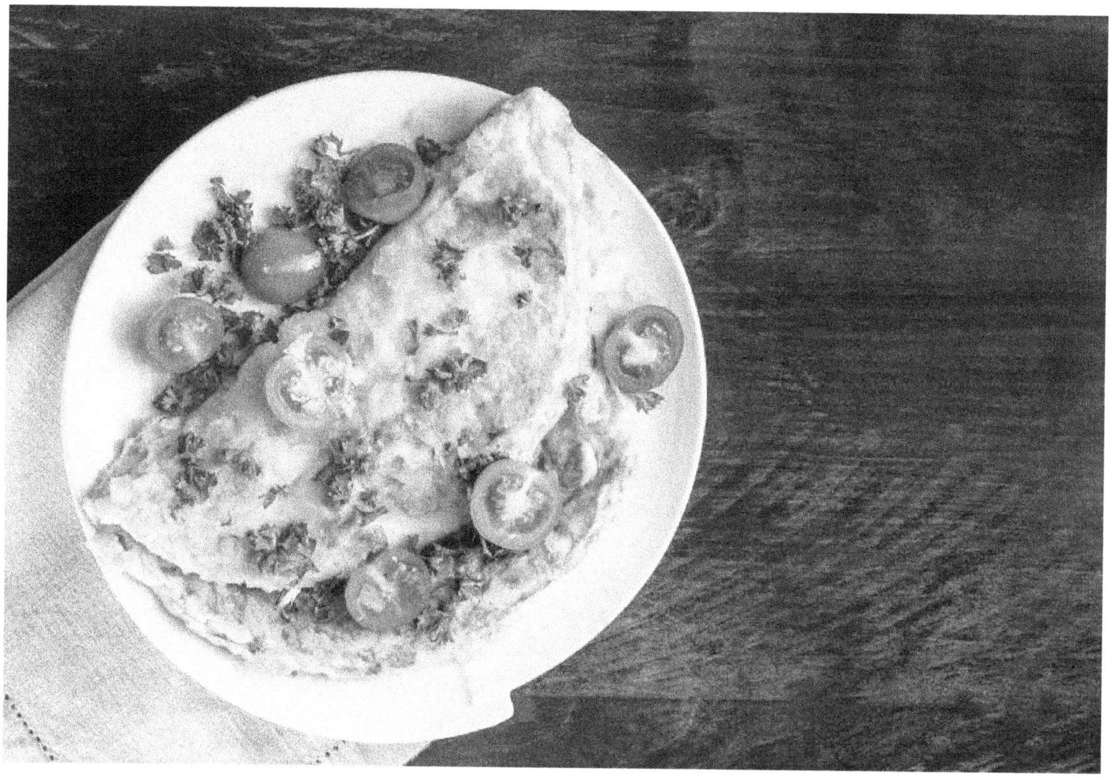

Dear, my readers. Thanks for your downloading this plant-based meal prep cookbook.

This cookbook offers a lot of insights and information into a plant-based diet. We have already made the research for you—all that you could ever want to know like insider knowledge. So, all you need to do is sit back, relax, read, and enjoy this new knowledge right at your fingertips. What's also nice about this eBook is that it couples the plant-based diet with meal prep.

A common factor why people fail to change their eating habits is the lack of preparation, busy lifestyle, and often once they fall off the track it's hard to find the motivation to get back on track. That is why, the best solution is to prepare ahead of time, during your off days from work. Place all your prepared food in meal prep containers for convenience. This book will help walk you through the basics of meal prepping with very helpful insider tips for you to start meal prepping like a pro.

I hope you will enjoy your journey to a healthier lifestyle with a plant-based diet through meal prepping as much as I have. Whether your goal is to lose weight or simply to embrace a healthier lifestyle—you have definitely picked the right book.

Enjoy and Good Luck!

Chapter 1 Plant-Based Diet: Your Guide to A Successful Plant-Based Diet

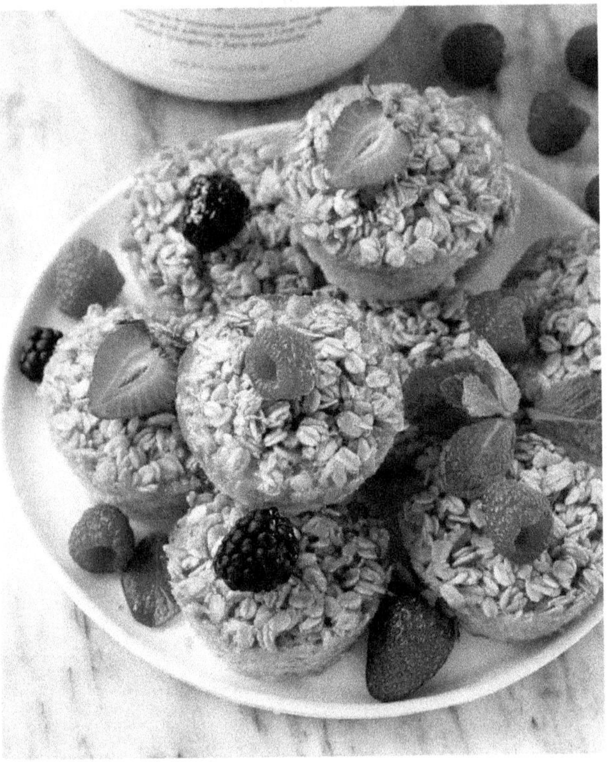

There are so many types of diets that are designed to help people maintain good health. In fact, there are so many arguments about which diet is the healthiest, but none is as healthy as the plant-based diet. I see a lot of people who suffer from lifestyle diseases such as hypertension, obesity, and diabetes who heavily rely on medications. While medication is good in maintaining stable vitals, didn't you know that these conditions are reversible as long as you live a healthy lifestyle? Many studies have shown that those who suffer from obesity, hypertension, and Type 2 diabetes can reverse their condition with a purely plant-based diet?

What Is A Plant-Based Diet?

There is no clear definition of what strictly a plant-based diet is all about. As the name implies, the plant-based diet emphasizes consuming only plant products such as vegetables, fruits, whole grain, seeds, nuts, and legumes. While the definition is simple enough, there are some variations of the plant-based diet and some variations exclude the consumption of refined food items like sugar, white flour, and processed oils. Another variation of the plant-based food is the exclusion of any kinds of oil or only consuming organic whole food plant-based ingredients. The thing is that whatever variation of the plant-based diet you adopt, you will be able to enjoy its many benefits.

The Benefits of Plant-Based Diet?

There are so many benefits of consuming a plant-based diet. This section will not only discuss the health benefits of the plant-based diet but also its many other advantages.

- May help maintain a healthy weight: Obesity is considered an epidemic in the United States. While many fad diets can facilitate weight loss, they do not have a lasting impact on weight loss. Many studies show that the high fiber content of a plant-based diet can be beneficial in weight loss and maintaining a healthy weight. When you adopt a plant-based diet, the kinds of foods that you also consume are not as calorie-dense compared to when you eat meat.
- Help maintain a healthy heart: Studies show that plant-based foods are rich in antioxidants and other phenolic compounds that are good in maintaining a healthy heart.

- **May reduce the risk for developing cancer:** Studies suggest that a plant-based diet may help reduce the risk of developing certain types of cancer particularly gastrointestinal cancer.
- **May reduce cognitive decline:** Diets rich in vegetables, fruits, and other plant-based ingredients can help reduce cognitive decline such as Alzheimer's disease due to its high number of plant compounds including antioxidants that can help protect brain cells against premature oxidation.
- **Help stabilize blood sugar levels:** The high fiber content of plant-based foods can help stabilize blood sugar levels as it takes longer for the body to process complex carbohydrates and turn it into glucose for the cells to use up. This prevents the upsurge of glucose in your blood that is characteristic of Type 2 Diabetes.
- **May help reduce greenhouse gas emissions:** Livestock production requires high water consumption and high greenhouse gas emissions. Growing plant ingredients require less water to produce therefore more sustainable. Unlike livestock, plant-based foods do not produce a lot of greenhouse gases. Studies show that the plant-based diet can reduce greenhouse gas emissions by as much as 70%.
- **A more sustainable method of growing food:** The plant-based diet encourages a more resilient and sustainable method of growing food. Not only are plant-based eaters concerned about not eating animal products, but they are also concerned with how their foods are grown. The rising movement of plant-based diet also increases the number of local farms growing produce in sustainable means.

Foods to Eat on A Plant-Based Diet

When you are about to make a switch to a plant-based diet, you need to understand the types of food that you need to eat to successfully follow this diet. Thus, below are the foods that you should consume when you follow this particular diet regimen:

- **Vegetables:** You are free to eat all types of vegetables there is as long as you don't have any allergic reactions to them. Make sure that you get enough green leafy vegetables in your diet as they are rich in antioxidants. Moreover, green leafy vegetables also contain substantial amounts of protein.
- **Fruits:** Consume fruits from all colors of the rainbow. It is important to take note that the more colorful the fruits are, the better it is for your body. Fruits are also a good source of natural sugars, so they are great alternatives especially if you are having some sweet cravings.
- **Starchy vegetables:** Starchy vegetables are calorie-dense, and it can provide you with enough energy to sustain your daily activities. Make sure that you opt for high fiber starchy vegetables such as sweet potatoes, taro, butternut squash, and cassava. If you opt for potatoes, make sure that you opt for boiled or steamed potatoes.
- **Healthy fats:** Healthy fats are good for the heart and these include avocados, olive oil, unprocessed coconut milk, and coconut oil.
- **Legumes:** Legumes such as peas, lentils, peanuts, beans, and chickpeas are good sources of plant protein. They are also calorie-dense thus it can help sustain your activities. You can also consume bean products such as tofu and tempeh as good sources of plant protein.
- **Whole grains:** Similar to starchy vegetables and legumes, whole grains are also calorie dense. However, make sure that you opt for whole grains because they contain complex carbohydrates that do not cause a spike in blood sugar levels. Examples of whole grains that you can consume include brown rice,

farro, rolled oats, brown rice pasta, red rice, black rice, barley, and rye to name a few.

- **Seeds and nuts:** Seeds and nuts are good sources of the anti-inflammatory Omega-3 fatty acid. Examples of seeds and nuts that you can consume while following this diet include almond, pistachios, cashews, sunflower seeds, sesame seeds, and many others. You can also use the seeds and nuts to make plant-based milk.
- **Spices and herbs:** Spices and herbs such as basil, turmeric, rosemary, and curry powder can help improve the flavor of your food. Moreover, they also come with health benefits as they contain high amounts of antioxidants.
- **Condiments:** You can also use a wide array of condiments to flavor your plant-based foods. These include mustard, soy sauce, nutritional yeast, vinegar, balsamic vinegar, and lemon juice.
- **Natural sweeteners:** Natural sweeteners such as date sugar and dried figs are good for those following the plant-based diet as they do not cause a spike on blood sugar level.
- **Beverages:** Beverages such as coffee, tea, and carbonated water are allowed in the plant-based diet.
- **Foods Not to Eat on A Plant-Based Diet**
- As there is no exact definition of the plant-based diet, the foods that you decide to avoid is definitely up to you. However, in a nutshell, there are certain foods that you certainly need to avoid while following the plant-based diet.
- **Fast food plant-based foods:** Fast food plant-based favorites such as oily fries and onion rings should be avoided as they are laden with trans-fat that are not good for the body.
- **Desserts and sweetened beverages:** Desserts are good as long as they are sweetened naturally. However, if they are sweetened by table sugar, then it may affect blood sugar levels. Avoid the consumption of commercial cookies, cereals, and others.
- **Refined grains:** Refined grains such as white rice, refined pasta, and white bread can cause a spike on blood sugar levels.

What about meat, dairy, and seafood? A plant-based diet does not simply mean eliminating animal products. Unlike the vegan diet, a plant-based diet is friendlier as it allows the consumption of lean sources of proteins on an occasional basis just to boost your body's level of Omega-3, Calcium, and Magnesium.

How to Transition to A Plant-Based Diet?

Transitioning to a plant-based diet is not as difficult as one might think. It may be challenging at first especially if you mostly consume meat, but it is, by no means, impossible to achieve. To be successful with your transition, there are certain things that you can do as follows:

- **Consume more veggies more often:** If you are strictly a meat eater, try to include more plant foods in your meals as much as you can.
- **Switch your portion sizes of meat to vegetables:** Slowly switch your meat portions to vegetables. You can do this in a staggered manner such that you can increase your consumption every week until you can easily adapt to the plant-based diet.
- **Eat more salad or vegetable soup before the main meal:** Eat more salad before the main meal so that you don't have to consume a lot of animal products when the main meal is served.
- **Plan your meals:** Planning your meals ahead of time is very important so that you don't have to eat something that you shouldn't. Making a meal plan can be challenging if you are new to the plant-based diet but there are so many online sources that can help you make exciting weekly meal plans so that you can eat delicious plant-based meals all the time.
- **Study restaurant menu:** If you are going out to eat at a restaurant, make sure that you study

the restaurant menu so that you don't order food that will keep you away from the plant-based diet.

- Considerations with The Plant-Based Diet
- When you are starting with a plant-based diet, there are certain things that you need to consider so that you will be able to follow this diet regimen long-term. Below are the things that you need to consider first when you follow the plant-based diet.
- Vitamin B12: Vitamin B12 is a very important nutrient for cell and blood health. Unfortunately, Vitamin B12 can only be sourced mostly from animal products. A deficiency of this vitamin can lead to nerve damage and anemia. People who consume mostly plants are at risk of developing Vitamin B12 deficiency. Consumption of B12 supplements or consuming food products that are fortified with Vitamin B12 is a good way to augment your body's requirement of this particular vitamin. You can also consume plant-based foods that are laden with B12 including nutritional yeast and some plant-based milk.
- Iron: Animal products, particularly red meat, are rich in iron. Iron is needed by the blood for proper transport of oxygen throughout the body. People who follow the plant-based diet may be at risk of iron deficiency. Moreover, iron has low bioavailability in plants. However, you can consume more plant-based foods rich in iron such as black beans, kidney beans, spinach, raisins, soybeans, cashews, tomato juice, and cabbages to name a few. Make sure that you consume citrus or other sources of Vitamin C as it increases the ability of your body to absorb iron.
- Protein: Protein is often associated with meat and people who consume little amount of meat may be deficient from protein. However, this is all a myth as people who follow the plant-based diet can source their protein from different kinds of foods particularly legumes. These include lentils, quinoa, beans, tofu, mushrooms, seeds, and nuts. Consuming proteins from a variety of plant foods can provide the necessary amino acids that the body can use for different physiological functions.
- Omega-3 fatty acids: Omega-3 fatty acids are often associated with deep-sea arctic fishes and they are good sources of DHA and EPA. This molecule is necessary as it protects the body against inflammation and cognitive decline. Although some plant-based foods such as flaxseed, hempseed, and walnuts contain the ALA type of Omega-3 fatty acid, it can be difficult for the body to convert it to EPA and DHA. People who are following the plant-based diet may want to supplement with Omega-3 tablets. There are plant-based Omega-3 fatty acids supplements that are available in the market. Moreover, dietitians also recommend people to reduce their consumption of linoleic acid sourced from sunflower oil, corn oil, and soybean oil as they may increase the inflammatory response of the body.

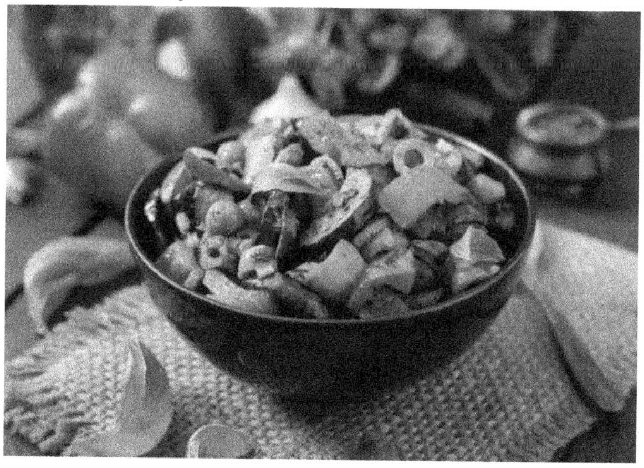

Takeaway

Consumption of foods that are higher in plant fibers can help improve health. Although it may be difficult to transition, it is not impossible to do so as long as you have the right guide. Let this book serve as your guide so that you will become successful in your transition to the plant-based diet.

Chapter 2 Meal Prepping Your Way to a Healthy Lifestyle

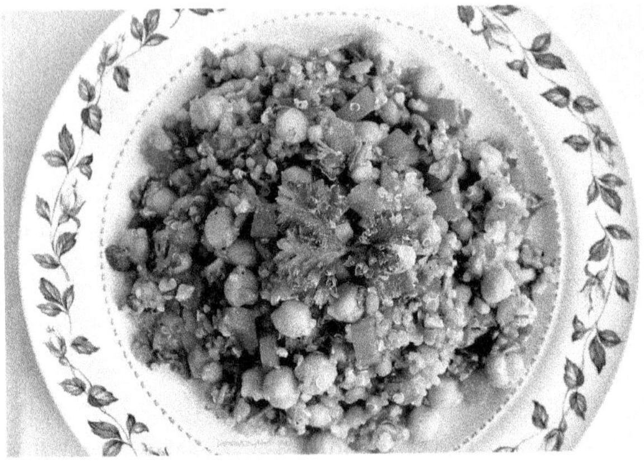

Many people are transitioning from meat-based diets today. The obvious alternatives to meat include nutritious vegetables, beans, and fruits, foods that are taken from plants. You don't have to worry too much about how to make delicious dishes if you plan your meals well. Taking time out to study your options will help you in this, but first, you should be able to know and define what a plant-based diet is based on a bit of history.

The definition of a plant-based diet can be one that is truly vegan, a dietary trend that has seen its ups and downs throughout history. The history of human eating habits had much to do with the capacity to gather food. The earliest form of food gathering meant months or seasons eating specific foods that were easy to gather in abundance. It didn't matter whether these were taken from animals or taken from plants, the main concern was that there was enough to eat.

Fast forward to today, where humans have the benefit of several thousand years of studying what is best to eat and developed complex economies based on agriculture, the science of farming or generating food in abundance. There are many opinions on this matter. Many believe that a true vegan diet is the best. Others say that they cannot do without meat. Good dietitians or expert nutritionists agree on one thing: balance.

Since we are here to help you plan, prepare, cook and store fresh, well-cooked meals that are mostly plant-based, we've cut down on the use of meat. This doesn't mean that meat is taken out of the picture entirely because we believe that meat is still a need in the human diet.

We have also studied the kind of diet in question with the following standards:

- The recipes used are based on good, practical nutrition.
- Meal servings are carefully set to provide just the right amounts of nutrients and calories.
- Emphasis is also made on using fresh, easy-to-find ingredients that are easy on the pocket.
- Preparation for and the storage of cooked meals were made with busy family life or professional in mind.

Nutritious eating is something that should be a habit for you. We believe that this is a primary need for maintaining good health. Also, we made sure that your meals would not be bland or boring. The recipes that you find here will be ones that you enjoy. Happy eating!

Prepping Your Plant-Based Meals

Welcome to the world of healthy eating–in the world of food, there are what you can call international recipes, the kinds of foods that have become widely available and eaten throughout the world. These might be tacos from Mexico, noodles from China or Japan, or pasta from Italy. These are some of the easiest to prepare meals and healthy ones at that, while you can be as flexible and creative as you want on the ingredients used and the way they are cooked and stored.

You don't have to be a trained chef or even a nutritionist to make these. Also, you needn't worry that you're serving will not be appreciated, since the recipes are based on popular dishes. Only the ingredients have been changed to accommodate more plant-based stuff. How the dishes taste was carefully tested before being included here. You won't find a marked difference between these dishes and those made with traditional portions of meat.

You'll become something of an expert on nutrition and cooking in the process, basically for your benefit and the benefit of your family or loved ones, your workmates or any small group you want to prepare food for. If you decide, you might even use these recipes for a small business you can moonlight in.

Prepping in this world is defined as a way to efficiently schedule your meal preparations so that you cut down on time and hassle. You can have well-cooked meals, say, prepared for a busy week. Shortcuts are made use of, which will also help you economize.

With our proven system, you can also say good-bye to grabbing unhealthy foods off store shelves, vending machines, or fast food restaurants on the run.

Advantages of Meal Preparation

You may already know some of these and may already have an idea based on what's already discussed. Meal prepping advantages will include:

- Savings – your food budget will stretch significantly once you get the hang of buying ingredients in bulk, which is cheaper, and dividing these for specific meals and days, which helps you cut down on wasted food.
- Good time management – it seems that every time you stand in front of the kitchen countertop or stove, you spend at least two hours to achieve anything. Carefully managed shortcuts will cut down the hours you spend each day preparing meals. The spare time you generate you can spend on quality activities or work.
- Eating healthier – where did this dream go to in your busy workday? Once you might have envisioned eating healthy with your family. Now's the time to do it!
- Reduce stress – your efforts in cooking up meals, even if well rewarded, shouldn't be stressful. Imagine coming home from work and stressing out on preparing a pasta dinner. Well planned and prepared meals will definitely reduce stress and give you happier mealtimes.
- Practice multitasking – you can become an expert multi-tasker in the kitchen in no time. Yes, you can get more out of your iPhone here by using it to keep notes, recorded recipes, advice and helps you surf the best recipes and tips online.
- Reduce overeating – unhealthy eating develops when portions are unregulated. A well-made portion for each person who will eat your meal means portions are controlled so that you eat enough calories, carbs, and nutrients. Plus, you'll add to savings and efficiency by not having leftovers to store or throw away.

Say Goodbye to Unwanted Ingredients and Chemicals in Your Food

We made sure that the recipes and ingredients are wholesome and organic, marketed with a minimum of preservatives, unpronounceable scientific names, and exotic ingredients on the nutrition table. They may come in mason jars, like pickles, fruit and vegetable preserves, with more natural preservatives. The ingredients will not have their nutritional value reduced to almost nil by over-processing.

Of course, some processing also helps you get better and cheaper foodstuffs. So, we carefully looked over those processed ingredients and used and chose those with the least amounts of stuff like "sodium", all forms of sodium. This element is something the body needs, too, but not in doses your body is unable to digest or wash out after each meal.

Homemade Foods Are A Preference

Added ingredients on frozen vegetables are avoided. Homemade is often best-made, and we can show you how to get more out of your food dollar by looking for the best and also the cheapest homemade stuff. Stores still offer some good things, but commercialization is double jeopardy you should do well to avoid most times.

This is what is called clean eating, and we provide helpful tips on how to thoroughly wash and prepare your food as well so that what you eat is the choice, not the unwanted, portions that come with organic or fresh foods. Preserved or processed foods, of course, have had these unwanted portions taken out, like stalks, roots, seeds, and skins.

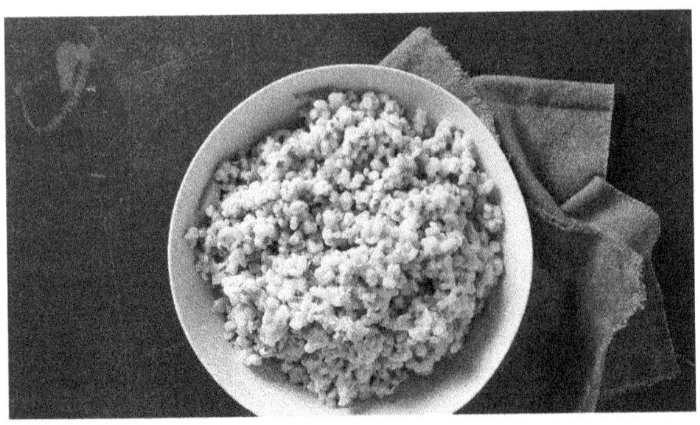

The Choicest Foods

The majority of what we have defined as a clean diet comes from plants. Although there may be other forms of nutritious diets, there is nothing known that can top fruits and vegetables. You will be enjoying the following mixture of plant-based foods and a selection of animal-based and processed products:

- Whole grains, nothing unprocessed – these include whole-wheat bread or pasta, brown or black rice, barley, and quinoa
- Green vegetables, root-based veggies, fruits, and some choice preserves
- Lean meat – these are lean ground pork, lamb or beef, and eggs, fish and
- seafood
- Some canned or preferably dry lentils, peas, beans (canned products either have no sodium or reduced-sodium additives)
- Dry roasted, saltless or raw nuts and their butter derivatives
- Soya based products
- Vegetable oils such as canola, olive, coconut, safflower and palm oil
- Nonfat or low-fat dairy products that include yogurt, milk, skimmed cheeses, cottage cheese
- Seeds (pumpkin, chia, flax, sesame, and others)

What to Expect in Your Recipes and Meal Plans?

Our recipes will have fruits like avocados and veggies like tomatoes taking center stage on the table. The most delicious recipes are actually those made from plant-based products, including spices and condiments. Of course, some spices are not used here, such as hot chilies, because they can cause heartburn.

If you have been used to eating unhealthy foods, you will appreciate the fact that you are eating delicious foods that you would not be guilty of eating. Again, we cannot overemphasize the use of those ingredients that do not cause any kind of discomfort or even long-term health effects.

There is minimal use of certain processed, packaged ingredients added to bigger portions of healthy ingredients. For instance, those recipes for dessert might have some commercial flour mixed in with flour made from whole grains. The following items are used minimally:

- Lard or any animal fat products
- Rich creams and dairy products like butter
- Foods that are fried
- Any full or whole cheese, milk, and ice cream
- Dark, rich chocolate
- Alcohol or and alcohol-based ingredients
- Any form of processed meat (i.e. sausages, hotdogs) but excluding nitrite-free products
- Juices made of 100% fruit

What You Will Not Miss

The foods that you have come to love or expect on meals that are high in saturated fat, sodium, and sugar will be things you would not miss, not if you expect to eat healthily. It might only be a force of habit for you to eat foods with these ingredients. The freshest, choicest ingredients enumerated in the earlier section will actually taste better than these.

These foods are among the most processed, meaning they have been cooked in a way that they no longer have nutrients. They might also contain an unhealthy amount of preservatives. We have avoided the following:

- Packaged easy-to-cook soups, or packaged pasta meals, other products full of additives, cholesterol, and sodium, and those that are too sweet
- Candy bars and commercial chocolate
- Baked goods that take longer to process, including cookies, donuts, and cakes
- Preserved fruits that go with thick syrups
- Ground pork in cans
- High energy or power drinks
- Carbonated beverages (i.e. sodas) and commercial beverages that are usually too sweet

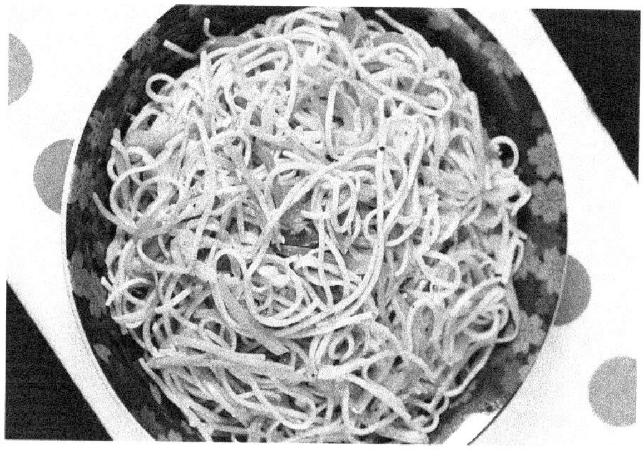

Recommended Dietary Guidelines

With the help of government agencies like the USDA and schools like the Harvard Medical School, nutritionists today know more about the precise portions that fulfill all of the body's needs for sustenance and overall health.

In this section, we will outline all the necessary food groups for a well-regulated diet that is mostly made up of plant-based foods. This is based on the daily recommended allowance of 2,000 calories.

Grains

Servings recommended: 1 ounce
Total daily intake: 6 ounces
Samples of 1-ounce servings:
1 slice whole-wheat bread
½ medium cup of pasta, cooked rice or cereal
1 medium cup cereal from a box
3 medium cups of commercial popcorn
1 small corn or flour tortilla
½ medium cup of pasta, cooked rice or cereal

Healthy Proteins

Servings recommended: ½ ounce
Total daily intake: 5 ounces
Sample servings:
2 servings of fish, lean beef or chicken breast
1 serving of any fresh nut or a mixture
1 tablespoon nut butter
1 large-sized egg
1 serving of seeds

Vegetables

Servings recommended:
Total daily intake: 2 ½ cups a day
Samples of 1 cup servings:
1 sweet potato (large, baked)
1 ear of corn (large)
1 potato (medium, baked)
1 cup of vegetables (like bell peppers, broccoli, squash, etc. which is either raw or cooked)
1 cup of vegetable juice (100% pure)
2 cups of leafy greens (recommended raw, like kale, collard greens, spinach, lettuce)

Nonfat or Low-fat Dairy

Daily serving recommended: 3 cups
Samples of 1 cup servings:
1 cup soya drink
1 ½ ounces Cheddar or Swiss cheese
1 ⅓ shredded part-skim mozzarella or equivalent
1 cup milk (nonfat or low-fat, skimmed is preferred)
2 cups cottage cheese (reduced-fat or nonfat)
1 cup yogurt (low-fat, Greek or traditional)

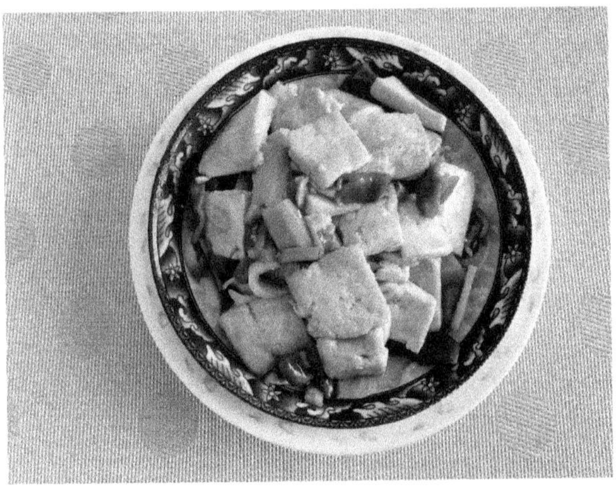

Fruits

Daily serving recommended: 3 cups
Samples of 1 cup servings:
1 cup of sliced fresh grapes, peaches, avocados, oranges, bananas
½ cup raisins or any dried fruit
30-35 grapes (seedless)
1 peach (large)
2-3 plums (medium)
8-10 strawberries (large)
1 cup fruit juice (apple or orange, 100% pure)

Oil Products

Daily Serving Recommended: 2-2 ½ tablespoons
Sample oils:
Corn, cottonseed, peanut, soya, sunflower, canola, olive and others

Preparing the Healthy Meal

You can mix and match the recommended foods and their servings. Be as creative as you can while keeping in mind that those that need more preparation should be prepared for and eaten on days that you are not too busy. The regimen may be a bit complicated at first, but once you get the hang of it, there is nothing easier.

Be prepared to think things over and "sacrifice" a few things. It's all a matter of adjustments and psychology. Your old habits, especially with regards to fast food or quickie alternatives, should be replaced by a balanced, nutritious and carefully prepared meal.

Prep Guidelines

- Start simply with some variety – during the first phase, the adjustment period, you must not stress out. The easiest meals to prepare should be your choice here. When you start rolling along, it would be easier to have some variety. Starting choices should be those recipes that are simpler to cook and with less use of ingredients and condiments. You can do this with pasta, for instance. Later on, with the basic preparation learned, you can add more spices, meats, cheese and so on.
- Learn to cook large amounts of food – also known as batch cooking, this is a key step in preparing meals for the entire week. Remember that you can freeze or refrigerate the cooked items, storing them in sealed containers, with labels for portions to be used

for each day of the week. You will spend less time worrying over the fire if the food is just right. Prepare the same ingredients such as meat or vegetables, which might be baked, boiled or steamed.

- **Reusing extra food** – this is another way of using your creativity. All the recipes included in the cookbook are basics that help you create many kinds of meals. You don't have to be bored or eat bland food. Sandwiches are a great way to reuse and economize. You probably do it all the time, and with the food you have, your sandwiches naturally become healthier.
- **Keep recipes easy and handy** – learning a few basic recipes is a way to be more efficient. Don't dream big or think of doing too much. This is not about a cooking competition but a lifestyle change. When you have mastered the easy and basic recipes, always keep the variants within easy reach so that you can buy up the ingredients you can plan ahead of time, from buying in bulk to storing your foods to batch cooking.
- **Use the most efficient storage containers** – there are several things to remember here. Common sense will tell you that great containers should be stackable or can be nested, will not leak, are safe for freezers, dishwashers, and the microwave. Also, keep up with the latest safe-for-food container materials that do not contain chemicals the FDA (Food and Drug Administration) has found to be hazardous to health.
- **Always remember to prioritize salads and vegetables** – in preparing meals for a week, make sure you have enough of these to last the entire time. Also, make sure that those items that are sensitive to moisture and the cold should be handled separately and put in special containers.
- **Keep track of the easier ingredients to have** – this is easy enough and should include preferred stuff, like potatoes or bananas. It all depends on you, but the recommendation to stock up on the foods listed earlier is also a good thing to follow. The easiest ingredients to have should also be found easily in stores in your neighborhood. Be aware of things like fruits in season or weather that can affect supplies of fish, for instance.

Your Sunday Best

The best day to prepare your meals for the week is Sunday, while you can use some hours on a Saturday if possible. Sundays mean being homebound, but this becomes more interesting with your focus on setting up the best meals possible for yourself or a group of persons or family.

Rope in anyone who can help, which should extend to the week, arranging schedules of who would do one thing while another does the next step. Children, for example, can participate with easy to do and remember tasks. This can also help you educate them on proper nutrition. Remember that the younger person is usually more interested in what they eat.

Don't use too much time, since longer hours can drag, and this means more mistakes in prepping meals. A good two hours of solid work should be spiced with some leisure activities or other errands or chores. A total of six hours can do for the entire day, spaced across morning, afternoon and early evening.

The 28 Days Meal Plan for Prepping

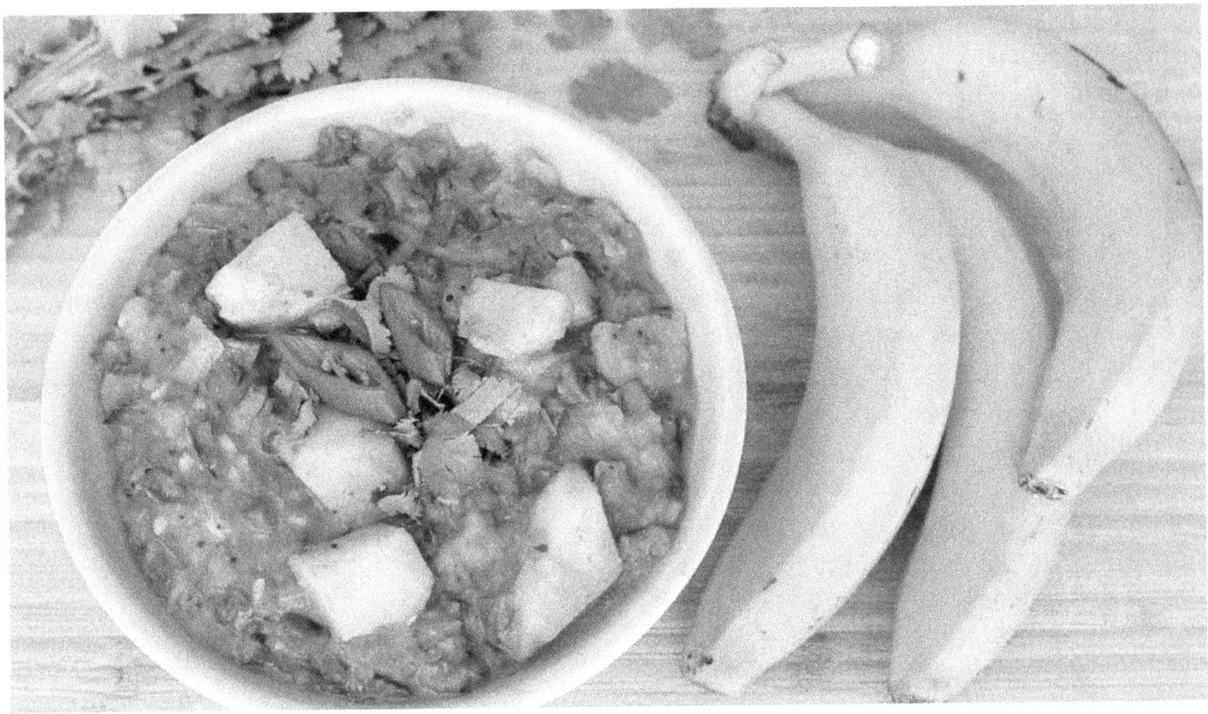

You can prepare a board for this, using basic recipes and variations with similar ingredients. Ask for suggestions from those who will eat the meals, since they might have preferences they can help prepare. It's all of a piece for a family to help each other out in preparing their meals for the week.

This can be a bonding process, too, or if you live as a couple or even alone, this will help you create more hours to spend outside or with friends. Again, the recommendation is to be creative as you can in the use of ingredients, in mixing and combining, in using variants or recipes and the like.

Meal Plan	Breakfast	Lunch	Dinner	Snacks/Dessert
Day-1	Veggie Omelet	Cauliflower with Peas	Mushroom Stew	Steamed Green Beans
Day-2	Veggies Quiche	Broccoli with Bell Pepper	Mixed Veggie Salad	Stir Fried Asparagus
Day-3	Simple Bread	Carrots with Snow Peas	Bell Pepper, Olives & Mushroom Stew	Roasted Brussels Sprout
Day-4	Quinoa Bread	Zucchini with Mushrooms	Farro & Zucchini Salad	Stir Fried Broccoli
Day-5	Fruity Oatmeal Muffins	Mushrooms Curry	Sweet Potato & Kale Stew	Sautéed Zucchini
Day-6	Oat Muffins	Banana Curry	Tofu & Veggies Salad	Soy Sauce Zucchini Noodles

Day-7	Tofu & Mushroom Muffins	Butternut Squash Curry	Cabbage & Broccoli Stew	Spiced Corn
Day-8	Coconut & Seeds Granola	Okra Curry	Chickpeas & Veggie Salad	Basil Cauliflower
Day-9	Nuts & Sees Granola	Spicy Veggies Combo	Lemony Veggie Stew	Sweet & Sour Kale
Day-10	Coconut Granola	Mixed Veggie Noodles	Chickpeas & Quinoa Salad	Nutty Spinach
Day-11	Veggie Omelet	Tempeh in Tomato Sauce	Tofu & Bell Pepper Stew	Garlicky Mushrooms
Day-12	Simple Bread	Tofu with Peas	Quinoa & Veggies Salad	Chocolate Cupcakes
Day-13	Coconut & Seeds Granola	Rice & Tofu Salad	Chickpeas Stew	Fruity Oat Bars
Day-14	Quinoa Bread	Kidney Beans & Pomegranate Salad	Beans & Couscous Salad	Chickpeas Fudge
Day-15	Fruity Oatmeal Muffins	Black Beans & Mango Salad	Beans & Pasta Stew	Oat Bars
Day-16	Oat Muffins	Beans & Corn Salad	Chickpeas & Lentil Salad	Apple Crisp
Day-17	Quinoa Bread	Mixed Grains Salad	Chickpeas & Veggie Stew	Blueberry Crumble
Day-18	Coconut Granola	Chickpeas & Lentil Salad	Mixed Grains Salad	Chocolate Cupcakes
Day-19	Nuts & Sees Granola	Beans & Couscous Salad	Barley & Lentils Stew	Stir Fried Asparagus
Day-20	Veggies Quiche	Quinoa & Veggies Salad	Beans & Corn Salad	Spiced Corn
Day-21	Coconut & Seeds Granola	Chickpeas & Quinoa Salad	Couscous Pilaf	Basil Cauliflower
Day-22	Tofu & Mushroom Muffins	Chickpeas & Veggie Salad	Corn & Veggie Salad	Fruity Oat Bars
Day-23	Oat Muffins	Farro & Zucchini Salad	Black-Eyed Peas Curry	Nutty Spinach
Day-24	Fruity Oatmeal Muffins	Tofu & Veggies Salad	Black Beans & Mango Salad	Basil Cauliflower
Day-25	Quinoa Bread	Mixed Veggie Salad	Mixed Grains Combo	Garlicky Mushrooms
Day-26	Simple Bread	Cauliflower with Peas	Kidney Beans & Pomegranate Salad	Roasted Brussels Sprout
Day-27	Veggies Quiche	Broccoli with Bell Pepper	Pasta with Asparagus	Chickpeas Fudge
Day-28	Veggie Omelet	Banana Curry	Oats Burgers	Basil Cauliflower

Chapter 3 Breakfast

Veggie Omelet

Prep time: 15 minutes, Cook time: 23 minutes; Serves 2

Ingredients:

- 8 ounces fresh asparagus, trimmed and cut into 1-inch pieces
- ¼ of red bell pepper, seeded
- ¼ of green bell pepper, seeded
- 1 tablespoon fresh chives, chopped
- ¾ cup water
- ½ cup superfine chickpea flour
- 1 tablespoon chia seeds
- 2 tablespoons nutritional yeast
- ½ teaspoon baking powder
- 1 teaspoon dried basil, crushed
- ¼ teaspoon ground turmeric
- ¼ teaspoon red pepper flakes, crushed
- Salt and ground black pepper, as required
- 1 small tomato, chopped

Instructions:

1. In a pan of the lightly salted boiling water, add the asparagus and cook for about 5-7 minutes or until crisp tender.
2. Drain the asparagus well and set aside.
3. Meanwhile, in a bowl, add the bell peppers, chives and water and mix.
4. In another bowl, add the remaining ingredients except tomato and mix well.
5. Add the water mixture into the bowl of flour mixture and mix until well combined.
6. Set aside for at least 10 minutes.
7. Lightly, grease a large nonstick skillet and heat over medium heat
8. Add ½ of the mixture and with the back of a spoon, smooth it.
9. Sprinkle half of the tomato over mixture evenly.
10. Cover the skillet tightly and cook for about 4 minutes.
11. Now, place half of cooked asparagus over one side of omelet.
12. Carefully, fold the other half over asparagus to cover it.
13. Cover the skillet and cook for 3-4 minutes more.
14. Repeat with the remaining mixture.
15. Serve warm.

Meal Prep Tip:

1. In a resealable plastic bag, place the cooled omelet slices and seal the bag.
2. Refrigerate for about 2-3 days.
3. Reheat in the microwave on High for about 1 minute before serving.

Nutrition Facts per Serving:

Calories: 271, Fats: 5.2g, Carbs: 44.7g, Fiber: 15.8g, Sugar: 9.5g, Proteins: 18.2g, Sodium: 104mg

Veggies Quiche

Prep time: 15 minutes, Cook time: 1 hour; Serves 4

Ingredients:

- 1 cup water
- Pinch of salt
- 1/3 cup bulgur wheat
- ¾ tablespoon light sesame oil
- 1½ cups fresh cremini mushrooms, sliced
- 2 cups fresh broccoli, chopped
- 1 yellow onion, chopped
- 16 ounces firm tofu, pressed and cubed
- ¾ tablespoon white miso
- 1¼ tablespoons tahini
- 1 tablespoon soy sauce

Instructions:

1. Preheat the oven to 350 degrees F. Grease a pie dish.
2. In a pan, add the water over medium heat and salt bring to a boil.
3. Stir in the bulgur and again bring to a boil.
4. Reduce the heat to low and simmer, covered for about 12-15 minutes or until all the liquid is absorbed.
5. Remove from the heat and let it cool slightly.
6. Now, place the cooked bulgur into the pie dish evenly and with your fingers, press into the bottom.
7. Bake for about 12 minutes.
8. Remove from the oven and let it cool slightly.
9. Meanwhile, in a skillet, heat oil over medium heat.
10. Add the mushrooms, broccoli and onion and cook for about 10 minutes, stirring occasionally.
11. Remove from the heat and transfer into a large bowl to cool slightly.
12. Meanwhile, in a food processor, add the remaining ingredients and pulse until smooth.
13. Transfer the tofu mixture into the bowl with veggie mixture and mix until well combined.
14. Place the veggie mixture over the baked crust evenly.
15. Bake for about 30 minutes or until top becomes golden brown.
16. Remove from the oven and set aside for at least 10 minutes.
17. With a sharp knife, cut into 4 equal sized slices and serve.

Meal Prep Tip:

1. In a reseal able plastic bag, place the cooled quiche slices and seal the bag.
2. Refrigerate for about 2-4 days.
3. Reheat in the microwave on High for about 1 minute before serving.

Nutrition Facts per Serving:

Calories: 212, Fats: 10.4g, Carbs: 19.6g, Fiber: 5.7g, Sugar: 3.4g, Proteins: 14.4g, Sodium: 425mg

Simple Bread

Prep time: 15 minutes, Cook time: 40 minutes; Serves 16

Ingredients:

- 2 teaspoons maple syrup
- 2 cups warm water
- 4 cups whole-wheat flour
- 1 tablespoon instant yeast
- ½ teaspoon salt

Instructions:

1. In a cup, dissolve the maple syrup in warm water.
2. In a large bowl, add the flour, yeast and salt and mix well.
3. Add the maple syrup mixture and mix until a sticky dough forms.
4. Transfer the dough into a greased 9×5-inch loaf pan.
5. Cover the loaf pan and set aside for about 20 minutes.
6. Preheat the oven to 390 degrees F.
7. Uncover the loaf pan and bake for about 40 minutes or until a toothpick inserted in the center comes out clean.
8. Remove the pan from oven and place onto a wire rack to cool for about 20 minutes.
9. Carefully, remove the bread from the loaf pan and place onto the wire rack to cool completely before slicing.
10. With a sharp knife, cut the bread loaf into desired sized slices and serve.

Meal Prep Tip:

1. In a resealable plastic bag, place the bread and seal the bag after squeezing out the excess air.
2. Keep the bread away from direct sunlight and preserve in a cool and dry place for about 1-2 days.

Nutrition Facts per Serving:

Calories: 118, Fats: 0.3g, Carbs: 24.7g, Fiber: 1g, Sugar: 0.6g, Proteins: 3.5g, Sodium: 76mg

Quinoa Bread

Prep time: 15 minutes, Cook time: 1½ hours; Serves 12

Ingredients:

- 1¾ cups uncooked quinoa, soaked overnight and rinsed
- ¼ cup chia seeds, soaked in ½ cup of water overnight
- ½ teaspoon bicarbonate soda
- Salt, as required
- ¼ cup olive oil
- ½ cup water
- 1 tablespoon fresh lemon juice

Instructions:

1. Preheat the oven to 320 degrees F. Line a loaf pan with parchment paper.
2. In a food processor, add all the ingredients and pulse for about 3 minutes.
3. Place the mixture into the prepared loaf pan evenly.
4. Bake for about 1½ hours or until a toothpick inserted in the center comes out clean.
5. Remove the pan from oven and place onto a wire rack to cool for about 20 minutes.
6. Carefully, remove the bread from the loaf pan and place onto the wire rack to cool completely before slicing.
7. With a sharp knife, cut the bread loaf into desired sized slices and serve.

Meal Prep Tip:

1. In a resealable plastic bag, place the bread and seal the bag after squeezing out the excess air.
2. Keep the bread away from direct sunlight and preserve in a cool and dry place for about 1-2 days.

Nutrition Facts per Serving:

Calories: 137, Fats: 6.5g, Carbs: 16.9g, Fiber: 2.6g, Sugar: 0g, Proteins: 4g, Sodium: 20mg

Fruity Oatmeal Muffins

Prep time: 15 minutes, Cook time: 20 minutes; Serves 6

Ingredients:

- ½ cup hot water
- ¼ cup ground flaxseeds
- 1 banana, peeled and sliced
- 1 apple, peeled, cored and chopped roughly
- 2 cups rolled oats
- ½ cup walnuts, chopped
- ½ cup raisins
- ¼ teaspoon baking soda
- 2 tablespoons ground cinnamon
- ½ cup almond milk
- ¼ cup maple syrup

Instructions:

1. Preheat the oven to 350 degrees F. Line a 12 cups muffin tin with paper liners.
2. In a bowl, add water and flaxseed and beat until well combined. Set aside for about 5 minutes.
3. In a blender, add the flaxseed mixture and remaining all ingredients except blueberries and pulse till smooth and creamy.
4. Transfer the mixture into prepared muffin cups evenly.
5. Bake for about 20 minutes or until a toothpick inserted in the center comes out clean.
6. Remove the muffin tin from oven and place onto a wire rack to cool for about 10 minutes.
7. Carefully invert the muffins onto the wire rack to cool completely before serving.

Meal Prep Tip:

1. Carefully invert the muffins onto a wire rack to cool completely.
2. Line 1-2 airtight containers with paper towels.
3. Arrange muffins over paper towel in a single layer.
4. Cover the muffins with another paper towel.
5. Refrigerate for about 2-3 days.
6. Reheat in the microwave on High for about 2 minutes before serving.

Nutrition Facts per Serving:

Calories: 351, Fats: 14.4g, Carbs: 51.8g, Fiber: 8.2g, Sugar: 22.4g, Proteins: 8.2g, Sodium: 61mg

Oat Muffins

Prep time: 15 minutes, Cook time: 20 minutes; Serves 6

Ingredients:

- ½ cup unsweetened almond milk
- 1 tablespoon apple cider vinegar
- 1½ cups whole-wheat flour
- 1 teaspoon baking powder
- 1 teaspoon baking soda
- ½ teaspoon ground cinnamon
- ¼ teaspoon ground nutmeg
- ¼ teaspoon ground ginger
- ½ teaspoon sea salt
- ½ cup unsweetened applesauce
- ½ cup maple syrup
- 1 teaspoon vanilla extract
- 1 cup carrots, peeled and grated
- ¼ cup walnuts, chopped
- ¼ cup raisins

Instructions:

1. Preheat the oven to 350 degrees F. Arrange a rack in the upper third of the oven. Grease a 12 cups muffin tin.
2. In a large bowl, add the almond milk and vinegar and mix well. Set aside.
3. In another large bowl, add the flour, baking powder, baking soda, spices and salt.
4. In the bowl of vinegar mixture, add the applesauce, maple syrup and vanilla extract and beat until well combined.
5. Add the flour mixture and mix until just combined.
6. Gently, fold in the carrots, walnuts and raisins.
7. Transfer the mixture into prepared muffin cups evenly and sprinkle with remaining oats.
8. Bake for about 17-20 minutes or until a toothpick inserted in the center comes out clean.
9. Remove from the oven and place the muffin tin onto a wire rack to cool for about 5 minutes.
10. Carefully invert the muffins onto the wire rack to cool completely before serving.

Meal Prep Tip:

1. Carefully invert the muffins onto a wire rack to cool completely.
2. Line 1-2 airtight containers with paper towels.
3. Arrange muffins over paper towel in a single layer.
4. Cover the muffins with another paper towel.
5. Refrigerate for about 2-3 days.
6. Reheat in the microwave on High for about 2 minutes before serving.

Nutrition Facts per Serving:

Calories: 257, Fats: 3.8g, Carbs: 51.8g, Fiber: 2.3g, Sugar: 22.4g, Proteins: 5g, Sodium: 399mg

Tofu & Mushroom Muffins

Prep time: 20 minutes, Cook time: 20 minutes; Serves 6

Ingredients:

- 1 teaspoon olive oil
- 1½ cups fresh mushrooms, chopped
- 1 scallion, chopped
- 1 teaspoon garlic, minced
- 1 teaspoon fresh rosemary, minced
- Ground black pepper, as required
- 1 (12.3-ounce) package lite firm silken tofu, drained
- ¼ cup unsweetened almond milk
- 2 tablespoons nutritional yeast
- 1 tablespoon arrowroot starch
- 1 teaspoon coconut oil, softened
- ¼ teaspoon ground turmeric

Instructions:

1. Preheat the oven to 375 degrees F. Grease a 12 cups of a muffin pan.
2. In a nonstick skillet, heat the oil over medium heat and sauté the scallion and garlic for about 1 minute.
3. Add the mushrooms and sauté for about 5-7 minutes.
4. Stir in the rosemary and black pepper and remove from the heat.
5. Set aside to cool slightly.
6. In a food processor, add the tofu and remaining ingredients and pulse until smooth.
7. Transfer the tofu mixture into a large bowl.
8. Fold in the mushroom mixture.
9. Place the mixture into prepared muffin cups evenly.
10. Bake for about 20-22 minutes or until a toothpick inserted in the center comes out clean.
11. Remove the muffin pan from the oven and place onto a wire rack to cool for about 10 minutes.
12. Carefully, invert the muffins onto wire rack and serve warm.

Meal Prep Tip:

1. Carefully invert the muffins onto a wire rack to cool completely.
2. Line 1-2 airtight containers with paper towels.
3. Arrange muffins over paper towel in a single layer.
4. Cover the muffins with another paper towel.
5. Refrigerate for about 2-3 days.
6. Reheat in the microwave on High for about 2 minutes before serving.

Nutrition Facts per Serving:

Calories: 74, Fats: 3.5g, Carbs: 5.3g, Fiber: 1.4g, Sugar: 1.1g, Proteins: 6.2g, Sodium: 32mg

Coconut & Seeds Granola

Prep time: 10 minutes, Cook time: 20 minutes; Serves 15

Ingredients:

- 3 cups unsweetened coconut flakes
- 1 cup walnuts, chopped
- ½ cup flaxseeds
- 2/3 cup pumpkin seeds
- 2/3 cup sunflower seeds
- ¼ cup coconut oil, melted
- 1 teaspoon ground ginger
- 1 teaspoon ground cinnamon
- 1/8 teaspoon ground cloves
- 1/8 teaspoon ground cardamom
- Pinch of salt

Instructions:

1. Preheat the oven to 350 degrees F. Lightly, grease a large rimmed baking sheet.
2. In a bowl, add the coconut flakes, walnuts, flaxseeds, pumpkin seeds, sunflower seeds, coconut oil, spices and salt and toss to coat well.
3. Transfer the mixture onto the prepared baking sheet and spread in an even layer.
4. Bake for about 20 minutes, stirring after every 3-4 minutes.
5. Remove the baking sheet from the oven and let the granola cool completely before serving.
6. Break the granola into desired sized chunks and serve with your favorite non-dairy milk.

Meal Prep Tip:

1. Transfer granola in an airtight container and store in a cool, dry place for up to 2 weeks.

Nutrition Facts per Serving:

Calories: 292, Fats: 26.4g, Carbs: 8.4g, Fiber: 5.3g, Sugar: 1.9g, Proteins: 6.2g, Sodium: 22mg

Nuts & Sees Granola

Prep time: 15 minutes, Cook time: 28 minutes; Serves 12

Ingredients:

- ½ cup unsweetened coconut flakes
- 1 cup raw almonds
- 1 cup raw cashews
- ¼ cup raw sunflower seeds, shelled
- ¼ cup raw pumpkin seeds, shelled
- ¼ cup coconut oil
- ½ cup maple syrup
- 1 teaspoon vanilla extract
- ½ cup golden raisins
- ½ cup black raisins
- Salt, as required

Instructions:

1. Preheat the oven to 275 degrees F. Line a large baking sheet with parchment paper.
2. In a food processor, add the coconut flakes, almonds, cashews and seeds and pulse until chopped finely.
3. Meanwhile, in a medium nonstick pan, add the oil, maple syrup and vanilla extract over medium-high heat and cook for about 3 minutes, stirring continuously.
4. Remove from the heat and immediately stir in the nuts mixture.
5. Transfer the mixture into the prepared baking sheet and spread evenly.
6. Bake for about 25 minutes, stirring twice.
7. Remove from the oven and immediately stir in the raisins.
8. Sprinkle with a little salt.
9. With the back of a spatula, flatten the surface of mixture.
10. Set aside to cool completely.
11. Then break into desired size chunks and serve with your choice of non-dairy milk and fruit's topping.

Meal Prep Tip:

1. Transfer granola in an airtight container and store in a cool, dry place for up to 2 weeks.

Nutrition Facts per Serving:

Calories: 237, Fats: 18.4g, Carbs: 25.5g, Fiber: 2.6g, Sugar: 16.3g, Proteins: 5g, Sodium: 18mg

Coconut Granola

Prep time: 10 minutes, Cook time: 18 minutes; Serves 4

Ingredients:

- 1 tablespoon coconut oil, melted
- 1 tablespoon coconut butter, melted
- 2-3 tablespoons maple syrup
- 1 teaspoon orange zest, grated freshly
- ½ teaspoon ground cinnamon
- Pinch of sea salt
- 2 cups coconut flakes

Instructions:

1. Preheat the oven to 350 degrees F. Line a cookie sheet with parchment paper.
2. In a bowl, mix together all ingredients except coconut flakes.
3. Spread coconut flakes in prepared cookie sheet.
4. Pour coconut oil mixture over flakes and gently, stir to mix.
5. Bake for about 12-15 minutes.
6. Remove from the oven and set aside to cool completely.
7. Then break into desired size chunks and serve with your choice of non-dairy milk and fruit's topping.

Meal Prep Tip:

1. Transfer granola in an airtight container and store in a cool, dry place for up to 2 weeks.

Nutrition Facts per Serving:

Calories: 221, Fats: 19g, Carbs: 14g, Fiber: 4.4g, Sugar: 8.7g, Proteins: 1.6g, Sodium: 69mg

Chapter 4 Soup and Stew

Mushroom Stew

Prep time: 15 minutes, Cook time: 15 minutes; Serves 4

Ingredients:

- 2 tablespoons olive oil
- 2 onions, chopped
- 3 garlic cloves, minced
- ½ pound fresh button mushrooms, chopped
- ¼ pound fresh shiitake mushrooms, chopped
- ¼ pound fresh Portobello mushrooms, chopped
- Salt and ground black pepper, as required
- ¼ cup homemade vegetable broth
- ½ cup coconut milk
- 2 scallions, chopped

Instructions:

1. In a large skillet, heat the oil over medium heat and sauté the onion and garlic for about 4-5 minutes.
2. Add the mushrooms, salt and black pepper and cook for about 4-5 minutes.
3. Add the broth and coconut milk and bring to a gentle boil.
4. Simmer for about 4-5 minutes or until desired doneness.
5. Stir in the scallion and remove from the heat.
6. Serve hot.

Meal Prep Tip:

1. Transfer the stew into a large bowl and set aside to cool.
2. Divide the stew into 4 airtight containers.
3. Cover and refrigerate for 1-2 days.
4. Reheat in the microwave before serving.

Nutrition Facts per Serving:

Calories: 182, Fats: 14.6g, Carbs: 12g, Fiber: 3.3g, Sugar: 5.6g, Proteins: 5.1g, Sodium: 87mg

Bell Pepper, Olives & Mushroom Stew

Prep time: 15 minutes, Cook time: 30 minutes; Serves 5

Ingredients:

- 3 tablespoons olive oil
- 1¼ pounds king oyster mushroom
- 1 red bell pepper, seeded and sliced
- 1 yellow bell pepper, seeded and sliced
- 1 red onion, chopped
- 4 garlic cloves, minced
- 10 green olives, pitted and sliced
- 6 ounces tomato paste
- 2¾ cups homemade vegetable broth
- 2 bay leaves
- Salt and ground black pepper, as required

Instructions:

1. In a large pan, heat the oil over medium-high heat and sauté the mushrooms, bell peppers, onions and garlic for about 5-6 minutes.
2. Stir in the olives, tomato paste, broth and bay leaves and bring to a boil.
3. Reduce the heat to low and simmer, covered for about 20 minutes or until desired doneness.
4. Season with the salt and black pepper and remove from the heat.
5. Serve hot.

Meal Prep Tip:

1. Transfer the stew into a large bowl and set aside to cool.
2. Divide the stew into 5 airtight containers.
3. Cover and refrigerate for 1-2 days.
4. Reheat in the microwave before serving.

Nutrition Facts per Serving:

Calories: 170, Fats: 10g, Carbs: 18.8g, Fiber: 4.5g, Sugar: 10.5g, Proteins: 6g, Sodium: 442mg

Sweet Potato & Kale Stew

Prep time: 15 minutes, Cook time: 30 minutes; Serves 8

Ingredients:

- 2 tablespoons canola oil
- 1 medium onion, chopped
- 2 large sweet potatoes, peeled and cut into ½-inch cubes
- 4 garlic cloves, minced
- 1 teaspoon fresh ginger, minced
- 1 Serrano pepper, seeded and chopped
- 1 tablespoon fresh thyme, chopped
- 1½ teaspoons curry powder
- 1½ teaspoons ground cumin
- ¼ teaspoon smoked paprika
- 2 cups tomatoes, chopped
- 3 cups water
- ½ cup peanuts, chopped
- 1/3 cup peanut butter
- 3 cups fresh kale, tough ends removed and chopped
- Salt and ground black pepper, as required
- ½ cup fresh cilantro, chopped

Instructions:

1. In a large pan, heat the oil over medium heat and sauté the onion, garlic, ginger and Serrano for about 5 minutes.
2. Add the sweet potato and sauté for about 3-4 minutes.
3. Stir in the thyme, curry powder, cumin and smoked paprika and sauté for about 1 minute.
4. Stir in the tomatoes and water and bring to a boil.
5. Reduce the heat to low and simmer, covered for about 5-10 minutes.
6. Stir in the chopped peanuts and peanut butter and simmer, uncovered for about 2-3 minutes.
7. Stir in the kale and simmer, uncovered for about 2-3 minutes.
8. Season with the salt and black pepper and remove from the heat.
9. Serve hot with the garnishing of cilantro.

Meal Prep Tip:

1. Transfer the stew into a large bowl and set aside to cool.
2. Divide the stew into 8 airtight containers.
3. Cover and refrigerate for 1-2 days.
4. Reheat in the microwave before serving.

Nutrition Facts per Serving:

Calories: 223, Fats: 13.8g, Carbs: 21.1g, Fiber: 4.6g, Sugar: 3.4g, Proteins: 7.2g, Sodium: 92mg

Cabbage & Broccoli Stew

Prep time: 15 minutes, Cook time: 35 minutes; Serves 4

Ingredients:

- 2 tablespoons olive oil
- 1 yellow onion, chopped
- 2 teaspoons fresh ginger, grated
- 1 teaspoon ground turmeric
- 1 teaspoon ground cumin
- Salt and ground black pepper, as required
- 1-2 cups water, divided
- 1 cup cabbage, shredded
- 1 cup broccoli, chopped
- 2 large carrots, peeled and sliced

Instructions:

1. In a large soup pan, heat the oil over medium heat and sauté onion for about 5 minutes.
2. Stir in the ginger and spices and sauté for about 1 minute.
3. Add 1 cup of water and bring to a boil.
4. Reduce the heat to medium-low and cook for about 10 minutes.
5. Add the vegetables and enough water that covers the half of vegetable mixture and stir to combine.
6. Increase the heat to medium-high and bring to a boil.
7. Reduce the heat to medium-low and cook, covered for about 10-15 minutes, stirring occasionally.
8. Serve hot.

Meal Prep Tip:

1. Transfer the stew into a large bowl and set aside to cool.
2. Divide the stew into 4 airtight containers.
3. Cover and refrigerate for 1-2 days.
4. Reheat in the microwave before serving.

Nutrition Facts per Serving:

Calories: 105, Fats: 7.4g, Carbs: 9.9g, Fiber: 2.8g, Sugar: 4g, Proteins: 1.7g, Sodium: 77mg

Lemony Veggie Stew

Prep time: 15 minutes, Cook time: 30 minutes; Serves 4

Ingredients:

- 2 tablespoons olive oil
- 1 large onion, chopped
- 2 garlic cloves, minced
- ¼ teaspoon fresh ginger, grated finely
- 1 teaspoon ground cumin
- 1 teaspoon cayenne pepper
- Salt and ground black pepper, as required
- 2 cups homemade vegetable broth
- 1½ cups small broccoli florets
- 1 cup cabbage, shredded
- 2 large carrots, peeled and sliced
- 1 tablespoon fresh lemon juice
- 1 teaspoon fresh lemon zest, grated finely

Instructions:

1. In a large soup pan, heat the oil over medium heat and sauté the onion for about 3-4 minutes.
2. Add the garlic, ginger and spices and sauté for about 1 minute.
3. Add 1 cup of broth and bring to a boil.
4. Add the vegetables and again bring to a boil.
5. Simmer, covered for about 15-20 minutes, stirring occasionally.
6. Stir in the lemon juice and remove from the heat.
7. Serve hot with the topping of lemon zest.

Meal Prep Tip:

1. Transfer the stew into a large bowl and set aside to cool.
2. Divide the stew into 4 airtight containers.
3. Cover and refrigerate for 1-2 days.
4. Reheat in the microwave before serving.

Nutrition Facts per Serving:

Calories: 121, Fats: 7.4g, Carbs: 13.1g, Fiber: 3.8, Sugar: 5.7g, Proteins: 2.2g, Sodium: 347mg

Tofu & Bell Pepper Stew

Prep time: 15 minutes, Cook time: 10 minutes; Serves 6

Ingredients:

- 2 tablespoons chile garlic sauce
- 1 jalapeño pepper, seeded and chopped
- 1 (16-ounce) jar roasted red peppers, rinsed and rinsed
- 2 cups homemade vegetable broth
- 2 cups water
- 1 medium red bell pepper, seeded and sliced thinly
- 1 medium green bell pepper, seeded and sliced thinly
- 1 (16-ounce) package extra-firm tofu, drained and cubed
- 1 (10-ounce) package frozen baby spinach, thawed

Instructions:

1. In a food processor, add chile garlic sauce, jalapeño pepper and roasted red peppers and pulse until a smooth puree forms.
2. In a large pan, add the puree, broth and water and mix well.
3. Place the pan over medium-high heat and bring to a boil.
4. Add the bell peppers and tofu and stir to combine.
5. Reduce the heat to medium and cook for about 5 minutes.
6. Stir in the spinach and cook for about 5 minutes.
7. Serve hot.

Meal Prep Tip:

1. Transfer the stew into a large bowl and set aside to cool.
2. Divide the stew into 6 airtight containers.
3. Cover and refrigerate for 1-2 days.
4. Reheat in the microwave before serving.

Nutrition Facts per Serving:

Calories: 121, Fats: 4.9g, Carbs: 12g, Fiber: 2.9g, Sugar: 6.8g, Proteins: 10.6g, Sodium: 442mg

Chickpeas Stew

Prep time: 15 minutes, Cook time: 35 minutes; Serves 3

Ingredients:

- 1 tablespoon olive oil
- 1 red bell pepper, seeded and julienned
- 3 scallions, sliced thinly
- 1 jalapeño pepper, chopped
- 2 garlic cloves, minced
- ½ teaspoon ground cumin
- ½ teaspoon paprika
- 4 cups tomatoes, crushed
- Salt and ground black pepper, as required
- ½ cup homemade vegetable broth
- 2 cups canned chickpeas
- 2 tablespoons fresh parsley, minced
- 1 teaspoon fresh lemon zest, grated

Instructions:

1. In a pan, heat the oil over medium heat and sauté the bell pepper, scallions, jalapeño, garlic, cumin and paprika for about 4-5 minutes.
2. Stir in the tomatoes, brown sugar, salt, black pepper and broth and simmer for about 20 minutes.
3. Stir in the chickpeas, parsley and lemon zest and simmer for about 10 minutes.
4. Serve hot.

Meal Prep Tip:

1. Transfer the stew into a large bowl and set aside to cool.
2. Divide the stew into 3 airtight containers.
3. Cover and refrigerate for 1-2 days.
4. Reheat in the microwave before serving.

Nutrition Facts per Serving:

Calories: 262, Fats: 8.4g, Carbs: 39.2g, Fiber: 12.3g, Sugar: 10.4g, Proteins: 12g, Sodium: 585mg

Beans & Pasta Stew

Prep time: 15 minutes, Cook time: 35 minutes; Serves 6

Ingredients:

- ¼ cup canola oil
- 1 large onion, chopped
- 8 ounces fresh shiitake mushrooms, sliced
- 1 medium tomato, chopped
- 2 tablespoons garlic, chopped finely
- 2 bay leaves
- 2 tablespoons mixed Italian herbs (rosemary, thyme, basil), chopped
- 1 teaspoon cayenne pepper
- 4 cups homemade vegetable broth
- 2 tablespoons apple cider vinegar
- 1 cup whole-wheat fusilli pasta
- 1/3 cup nutritional yeast
- 1/3 cup roasted tomato salsa
- 8 ounces fresh collard greens
- 1 (15-ounce) can cannellini beans, rinsed and drained
- Salt and ground black pepper, as required

Instructions:

1. In a large pan, heat the oil over medium heat and sauté the onion, mushrooms, potato and tomato for about 4-5 minutes.
2. Add the garlic, bay leaves, herbs and cayenne pepper and sauté for about 1 minute.
3. Add the broth and bring to a boil.
4. Stir in the vinegar, pasta, nutritional yeast and tomato salsa and again bring to a boil.
5. Reduce the heat to medium-low and simmer, covered for about 20 minutes.
6. Uncover and stir in the greens and beans.
7. Simmer for about 4-5 minutes.
8. Stir in the salt and black pepper and remove from the heat.
9. Serve hot.

Meal Prep Tip:

1. Transfer the stew into a large bowl and set aside to cool.
2. Divide the stew into 6 airtight containers.
3. Cover and refrigerate for 1-2 days.
4. Reheat in the microwave before serving.

Nutrition Facts per Serving:

Calories: 254, Fats: 11.1g, Carbs: 28.4g, Fiber: 11.7g, Sugar: 3.9g, Proteins: 14.4g, Sodium: 737mg

Chickpeas & Veggie Stew

Prep time: 15 minutes, Cook time: 40 minutes; Serves 6

Ingredients:

- 1 tablespoon olive oil
- 1 medium sweet onion, chopped
- ½ teaspoons fresh ginger, grated
- 2 garlic cloves, minced
- ¼ teaspoon ground cumin
- ¾ teaspoon ground cinnamon
- 1-2 teaspoons red chili flakes, crushed
- 3½ cups butternut squash, peeled and chopped
- Salt and ground black pepper, as required
- 1½ cups water, divided
- ¼ cup creamy natural almond butter
- 1½ cups cooked chickpeas
- 3 cups fresh kale, trimmed and chopped
- ½ cup raw almonds, chopped

Instructions:

1. In a large soup pan, heat oil over medium heat and cook onion, covered for about 5 minutes, stirring occasionally.
2. Stir in ginger, garlic and spices and sauté for about 1 minute.
3. Add squash and stir to combine well.
4. Add 1¼ cups of water, salt and black pepper and bring to a boil.
5. Reduce the heat to low.
6. In a bowl, mix together remaining water and peanut butter.
7. Add peanut butter mixture in pan and stir to combine.
8. Simmer, covered for about 20 minutes.
9. Stir in chickpeas, kale and almonds and simmer for about 10 minutes more.
10. Remove from the heat and serve hot.

Meal Prep Tip:

1. Transfer the stew into a large bowl and set aside to cool.
2. Divide the stew into 6 airtight containers.
3. Cover and refrigerate for 1-2 days.
4. Reheat in the microwave before serving.

Nutrition Facts per Serving:

Calories: 186, Fats: 7.6g, Carbs: 25.8g, Fiber: 5.5g, Sugar: 3.2g, Proteins: 6.7g, Sodium: 145mg

Barley & Lentils Stew

Prep time: 20 minutes, Cook time: 50 minutes; Serves 8

Ingredients:

- 2 tablespoons olive oil
- 2 carrots, peeled and chopped
- 1 large onion, chopped
- 2 celery stalks, chopped
- 2 garlic cloves, minced
- 1 teaspoon ground coriander
- 2 teaspoons ground cumin
- 1 teaspoon cayenne pepper
- 1 cup barley
- 1 cup red lentils
- 5 cups tomatoes, chopped finely
- 5-6 cups homemade vegetable broth
- 6 cups fresh spinach, torn
- Salt and ground black pepper, as required

Instructions:

1. In a large pan, heat the oil over medium heat and sauté the carrots, onion, celery and celery for about 5 minutes.
2. Add the garlic and spices and sauté for about 1 minute.
3. Add the barley, lentils, tomatoes and broth and bring to a boil.
4. Reduce the heat to low and simmer, covered for about 40 minutes.
5. Stir in the spinach, salt and black pepper and simmer for about 3-4 minutes.
6. Serve hot.

Meal Prep Tip:

1. Transfer the stew into a large bowl and set aside to cool.
2. Divide the stew into 8 airtight containers.
3. Cover and refrigerate for 1-2 days.
4. Reheat in the microwave before serving.

Nutrition Facts per Serving:

Calories: 264, Fats: 5.7g, Carbs: 41.1g, Fiber: 14.1g, Sugar: 5.8g, Proteins: 14.3g, Sodium: 540mg

Chapter 5 Beans and Grains

Couscous Pilaf

Prep time: 20 minutes, Cook time: 22 minutes; Serves 4

Ingredients:

- 3 tablespoons vegetable oil
- 1 medium onion, chopped
- 1 medium parsnip, peeled and sliced thinly
- 1 medium carrot, peeled and sliced thinly
- 1 medium zucchini, cut into ¾-inch pieces
- 1 medium yellow squash, cut into ¾-inch pieces
- 2 garlic cloves, minced
- 1 teaspoon ground cumin
- ½ teaspoon red pepper flakes, crushed
- ½ teaspoon smoked paprika
- 1½ cups couscous
- Salt and ground black pepper, as required
- ½ cup dried apricots, chopped
- 2¼ cups homemade vegetable broth
- ¼ cup fresh cilantro, chopped
- ½ cup almonds, toasted and chopped

Instructions:

1. In a large cast iron skillet, heat the oil over medium-high heat and sauté the onion for about 4-5 minutes.
2. Add the parsnip and carrot and sauté for about 4-5 minutes.
3. Add the zucchini, yellow squash, garlic and spices and sauté for about 4-5 minutes.
4. Stir in the couscous and cook for about 2 minutes, stirring occasionally.
5. Stir in the apricots and broth and cook, covered for about 5 minutes or until all the liquid is absorbed.
6. Remove from the heat and with a fork, fluff the couscous completely.
7. Stir in the cilantro and almonds and serve.

Meal Prep Tip:

1. Transfer the couscous mixture into a large bowl and set aside to cool.
2. Divide the mixture into 4 airtight containers.
3. Cover and refrigerate for 2 days.
4. Reheat in the microwave before serving.

Nutrition Facts per Serving:

Calories: 484, Fats:17.2g, Carbs: 71g, Fiber: 9.6g, Sugar: 0.6g, Proteins: 13.3g, Sodium: 370mg

Black-Eyed Peas Curry

Prep time: 15 minutes, Cook time: 15 minutes; Serves 3

Ingredients:

- 1 teaspoon canola oil
- 1 red bell pepper, seeded and chopped
- ¼ cup shallot, chopped
- 2 teaspoons fresh ginger, minced
- 3 garlic cloves, minced
- 1 fresh green chili, chopped finely
- 1 tablespoon fresh thyme, chopped
- 2 bay leaves
- 2 teaspoons curry powder
- ½ teaspoon ground cumin
- 1 (16-ounce) can black-eyed peas, drained and rinsed
- ¾ cup water
- ¾ cup coconut milk
- 1 teaspoon unsweetened applesauce
- 1 tablespoon fresh lime juice
- Salt and ground black pepper, as required
- 2 tablespoons fresh parsley, chopped

Instructions:

1. In a pan, heat the oil over medium heat and sauté the bell pepper and shallot for about 4-5 minutes.
2. Add the ginger, garlic, green chili, thyme, bay leaves, curry powder and cumin and sauté for about 1 minute.
3. Add the black-eyed peas, water, coconut milk and applesauce and bring to a boil.
4. Cover and cook for about 5 minutes.
5. Stir in the lime juice, salt and black pepper and cook or about 1 minute.
6. Remove from the heat and discard the bay leaves.
7. Serve hot with the garnishing of parsley.

Meal Prep Tip:

1. Transfer the black-eyed peas mixture into a large bowl and set aside to cool.
2. Divide the mixture into 3 airtight containers.
3. Cover and refrigerate for 2 days.
4. Reheat in the microwave before serving.

Nutrition Facts per Serving:

Calories: 305, Fats: 17.6g, Carbs: 32.3g, Fiber: 8g, Sugar: 4.3g, Proteins: 10.2g, Sodium: 99mg

Mixed Grains Combo

Prep time: 15 minutes, Cook time: 30 minutes; Serves 6

Ingredients:

- ¾ cup amaranth
- 1 cup quinoa
- ¼ cup wild rice
- 4¼ cups water
- 2 teaspoons ground cumin
- ½ teaspoon paprika
- Salt, as required
- 1 cup canned chickpeas, drained and rinsed
- ½ cup raisins
- 2 medium carrots, peeled and grated
- 1 garlic clove, minced
- Salt and ground black pepper, as required

Instructions:

1. In a large pan, add the amaranth, quinoa, wild rice, water and spices over medium-high heat and bring to a boil.
2. Reduce the heat to medium-low and simmer, covered for about 20-25 minutes.
3. Stir in remaining ingredients and simmer for about 3-5 minutes.
4. Remove from the heat and serve.

Meal Prep Tip:

1. Transfer the grains mixture into a large bowl and set aside to cool.
2. Divide the mixture into 6 airtight containers.
3. Cover and refrigerate for 2 days.
4. Reheat in the microwave before serving.

Nutrition Facts per Serving:

Calories: 311, Fats: 3.9g, Carbs: 58.5g, Fiber: 7.4g, Sugar: 8.8g, Proteins: 11.6g, Sodium: 61mg

Pasta with Asparagus

Prep time: 15 minutes, Cook time: 12 minutes; Serves 6

Ingredients:

- ¼ cup olive oil
- 5 garlic cloves, minced
- ½ teaspoon red pepper flakes, crushed
- 1/8 teaspoon hot pepper sauce
- 1 pound fresh asparagus, trimmed and cut into 1½-inch pieces
- Salt and ground black pepper, as required
- ½ pound cooked whole-wheat pasta, drained

Instructions:

1. In a large cast-iron skillet, heat the oil over medium heat and cook the garlic, red pepper flakes and hot pepper sauce for about 1 minute.
2. Add the asparagus, salt and black pepper and cook for about 8-10 minutes, stirring occasionally.
3. Add the hot pasta and toss to coat well.
4. Serve immediately.

Meal Prep Tip:

1. Transfer the pasta mixture into a large bowl and set aside to cool.
2. Divide the mixture into 6 airtight containers.
3. Cover and refrigerate for 2 days.
4. Reheat in the microwave before serving.

Nutrition Facts per Serving:

Calories: 233, Fats: 9.3g, Carbs: 32.2g, Fiber: 3g, Sugar: 1.5g, Proteins: 7.2g, Sodium: 33mg

Oats Burgers

Prep time: 15 minutes, Cook time: 20 minutes; Serves 4

Ingredients:

- 1 pound firm tofu, pressed and crumbled
- ¾ cup rolled oats
- ¼ cup flaxseeds
- 1 medium onion, chopped finely
- 2 cups frozen spinach, thawed and squeezed
- 2 garlic cloves, minced
- 1 jalapeño pepper, seeded and minced
- 1 teaspoon ground cumin
- ½ teaspoon red pepper flakes, crushed
- Salt and ground black pepper, as required
- 2 tablespoons extra-virgin olive oil

Instructions:

1. In a large bowl, add all the ingredients except oil and salad greens and mix until well combined.
2. Set aside for about 10 minutes.
3. Make 4 equal sized patties from the mixture.
4. In a nonstick frying pan, heat the oil over medium heat and cook the patties for about 8-10 minutes per side.
5. Serve hot.

Meal Prep Tip:

1. Remove the patties from heat and set aside to cool completely.
2. Store in an airtight container, by placing parchment papers between the burgers to avoid the sticking.
3. These burgers can be stored in the freezer for up to 3 weeks.
4. Before serving, thaw the burgers and then reheat in microwave.

Nutrition Facts per Serving:

Calories: 255, Fats: 15.2g, Carbs: 18.5g, Fiber: 5.6g, Sugar: 2.3g, Proteins: 136g, Sodium: 70mg

Chickpeas & Couscous Burgers

Prep time: 20 minutes, Cook time: 1 hour; Serves 4

Ingredients:

- 1 cup water
- 1/3 cup dry couscous
- 1½ cups broccoli florets
- 2 teaspoons olive oil
- ½ cup onion, chopped
- ½ cup scallion, chopped
- 2 teaspoons ground cumin
- 1 tablespoon sesame tahini
- 1 (15-ounce) can chickpeas, rinsed and drained
- ½ cup whole-wheat breadcrumbs

Instructions:

1. Preheat the oven to 400 degrees F. Line a baking sheet with a piece of foil.
2. In a small pan, mix together the water and couscous over medium heat and bring to a boil.
3. Immediately, remove from the heat and set aside for about 10 minutes or until all the liquid is absorbed.
4. Meanwhile, in a pan of the boiling water, arrange a steamer basket.
5. Place the broccoli in steamer basket and steam, covered for about 5-7 minutes.
6. Drain the broccoli well.
7. Meanwhile, in a skillet, heat the oil over medium heat and sauté the onion and scallion for about 3-5 minutes.
8. Stir in the cumin and immediately remove from the heat.
9. In a food processor, add the couscous, broccoli, onion mixture, tahini and chickpeas and pulse until well combined.
10. Transfer the mixture into a bowl.
11. Add the breadcrumbs and stir to combine.
12. Make 4 equal sized patties from the mixture.
13. Arrange the patties onto the prepared baking sheet in a single layer.
14. Bake for about 50 minutes, flipping once halfway through.
15. Serve hot.

Meal Prep Tip:

1. Remove the patties from heat and set aside to cool completely.
2. Store in an airtight container, by placing parchment papers between the burgers to avoid the sticking.
3. These burgers can be stored in the freezer for up to 3 weeks.
4. Before serving, thaw the burgers and then reheat in microwave.

Nutrition Facts per Serving:

Calories: 292, Fats: 6.9g, Carbs: 44.8g, Fiber: 7.8g, Sugar: 2.3g, Proteins: 12.2g, Sodium: 146mg

Black Beans Burgers

Prep time: 20 minutes, Cook time: 45 minutes; Serves 6

Ingredients:

- ½ cup walnuts
- 1 carrot, peeled and chopped
- 1 celery stalk, chopped
- 4 scallions, chopped
- 5 garlic cloves, chopped
- 2¼ cups cooked black beans
- 2½ cups sweet potato, peeled and grated
- ½ teaspoon red pepper flakes, crushed
- Salt and ground black pepper, as required

Instructions:

1. Preheat the oven to 400 degrees F. Line a baking sheet with parchment paper.
2. In a food processor, add the walnuts and pulse until grounded finely.
3. Add the carrot, celery, scallion and garlic and pulse until chopped finely.
4. Transfer the vegetable mixture into a large bowl.
5. In the same food processor, add the beans and pulse until chopped.
6. Add 1½ cups of sweet potato and pulse until a chunky mixture forms.
7. Transfer the bean mixture into the bowl with vegetable mixture.
8. Stir in remaining sweet potato and spices and mix until well combined.
9. Make 8 equal sized patties from the mixture.
10. Arrange the patties onto the prepared baking sheet in a single layer.
11. Bake for about 25 minutes.
12. Serve hot.

Meal Prep Tip:

1. Remove the patties from heat and set aside to cool completely.
2. Store in an airtight container, by placing parchment papers between the burgers to avoid the sticking.
3. These burgers can be stored in the freezer for up to 3 weeks.
4. Before serving, thaw the burgers and then reheat in microwave.

Nutrition Facts per Serving:

Calories: 234, Fats: 7.1g, Carbs: 34.5g, Fiber: 8.6g, Sugar: 6.3g, Proteins: 9.9g, Sodium: 80mg

Chapter 6 Vegetable Recipes

Cauliflower with Peas

Prep time: 15 minutes, Cook time: 15 minutes; Serves 3

Ingredients:

- ¼ cup water
- 2 medium tomatoes, chopped
- 2 tablespoons olive oil
- 3 medium garlic cloves, minced
- ½ tablespoon fresh ginger, minced
- 1 teaspoon ground cumin
- 2 teaspoons ground coriander
- 1 teaspoon cayenne pepper
- ¼ teaspoon ground turmeric
- 2 cups cauliflower, chopped
- 1 cup fresh green peas, shelled
- Salt and ground black pepper, as required
- ½ cup warm water

Instructions:

1. In a blender, add tomato and ¼ cup of water and pulse until a smooth puree forms. Set aside.
2. In a large skillet, heat the oil over medium heat and sauté the garlic, ginger, green chilies and spices for about 1 minute.
3. Add the cauliflower, peas and tomato puree and cook, stirring for about 3-4 minutes.
4. Add the warm water and bring to a boil.
5. Reduce the heat to medium-low and cook, covered for about 8-10 minutes or until vegetables are done completely.
6. Serve hot.

Meal Prep Tip:

1. Transfer the veggie mixture into a large bowl and set aside to cool.
2. Divide the mixture into 3 airtight containers.
3. Cover and refrigerate for 2 days.
4. Reheat in the microwave before serving.

Nutrition Facts per Serving:

Calories: 163, Fats: 10.1g, Carbs: 16.1g, Fiber: 5.6g, Sugar: 6.7g, Proteins: 5.1g, Sodium: 80mg

Broccoli with Bell Pepper

Prep time: 15 minutes, Cook time: 20 minutes; Serves 3

Ingredients:

- 2 tablespoons olive oil
- 2 medium garlic cloves, minced
- 1½ cups red bell pepper, seeded and sliced
- 1½ cups small broccoli florets
- ¼ cup soy sauce
- Freshly ground black pepper, as required
- 1 tablespoon white sesame seeds

Instructions:

1. In a large skillet, heat the oil over medium-high heat and sauté the garlic for about 1 minute.
2. Add the vegetables and cook for about 5-6 minutes.
3. Add the soy sauce and cook for about 2-3 minutes.
4. Season with black pepper and remove from heat.
5. Serve hot with the garnishing of sesame seeds.

Meal Prep Tip:

1. Transfer the veggie mixture into a large bowl and set aside to cool.
2. Divide the mixture into 3 airtight containers.
3. Cover and refrigerate for 2 days.
4. Reheat in the microwave before serving.

Nutrition Facts per Serving:

Calories: 144, Fats: 11.2g, Carbs: 10.5g, Fiber: 2.5g, Sugar: 4.2g, Proteins: 3.8g, Sodium: 1200mg

Carrots with Snow Peas

Prep time: 15 minutes, Cook time: 6 minutes; Serves 4

Ingredients:

- 2 tablespoons olive oil
- 1¾ cups sliced fresh carrots
- 2¾ cups fresh snow peas
- 1 shallot, minced
- Salt, as required
- 1 tablespoon vegetable broth

Instructions:

1. In a large cast iron skillet, melt the butter over medium heat and stir fry the carrots for about 3 minutes
2. Add the snow peas, shallot and salt and stir fry for about 2 minutes.
3. Stir in the broth and stir fry for about 1 minute.
4. Remove from the heat and serve hot.

Meal Prep Tip:

1. Transfer the veggie mixture into a large bowl and set aside to cool.
2. Divide the mixture into 4 airtight containers.
3. Cover and refrigerate for 2 days.
4. Reheat in the microwave before serving.

Nutrition Facts per Serving:

Calories: 129, Fats: 7.3g, Carbs: 13.3g, Fiber: 4.3g, Sugar: 6.8g, Proteins: 4.1g, Sodium: 85mg

Zucchini with Mushrooms

Prep time: 15 minutes, Cook time: 12 minutes; Serves 4

Ingredients:

- 2 tablespoons coconut oil
- ½ pound fresh mushrooms, sliced
- Salt and ground black pepper, as required
- 3 garlic cloves, minced
- 1 Serrano pepper, chopped
- 4 scallions, chopped
- 2 pounds zucchini, halved lengthwise and sliced
- ¼ cup fresh parsley, chopped

Instructions:

1. In a large skillet, melt the coconut oil over medium-high heat and stir fry the mushrooms for about 5-6 minutes.
2. With a slotted spoon, transfer the mushrooms into bowl.
3. In the same skillet, add the garlic, Serrano pepper and scallion over medium heat and sauté for about 1 minute.
4. Add the zucchini and stir fry for about 2-3 minutes.
5. Stir in the mushrooms and cook for about 1-2 minutes.
6. Stir in the parsley and remove from heat.
7. Serve hot.

Meal Prep Tip:

1. Transfer the veggie mixture into a large bowl and set aside to cool.
2. Divide the mixture into 4 airtight containers.
3. Cover and refrigerate for 2 days.
4. Reheat in the microwave before serving.

Nutrition Facts per Serving:

Calories: 117, Fats: 7.5g, Carbs: 11.6g, Fiber: 3.7g, Sugar: 5.4g, Proteins: 5.1g, Sodium: 70mg

Mushrooms Curry

Prep time: 15 minutes, Cook time: 20 minutes; Serves 3

Ingredients:

- 2 cups tomatoes, chopped
- 1 green chili, chopped
- 1 teaspoon fresh ginger, chopped
- ¼ cup cashews
- 2 tablespoons canola oil
- ½ teaspoon cumin seeds
- ¼ teaspoon ground coriander
- ¼ teaspoon ground turmeric
- ¼ teaspoon red chili powder
- 1½ cups fresh shiitake mushrooms, sliced
- 1½ cups fresh button mushrooms, sliced
- 1 cup frozen corn kernels
- 1¼ cups water
- ¼ cup coconut milk
- Salt and ground black pepper, as required

Instructions:

1. In a food processor, add the tomatoes, green chili, ginger and cashews and pulse until a smooth paste forms.
2. In a pan, heat the oil over medium heat and sauté the cumin seeds for about 1 minute.
3. Add the spices and sauté for about 1 minute.
4. Add the tomato paste and cook for about 5 minutes.
5. Stir in the mushrooms, corns, water and coconut milk and bring to a boil.
6. Cook for about 10-12 minutes, stirring occasionally.
7. Season with the salt and black pepper and remove from the heat.
8. Serve hot.

Meal Prep Tip:

1. Transfer the curry into a large bowl and set aside to cool.
2. Divide the mixture into 3 airtight containers.
3. Cover and refrigerate for 2 days.
4. Reheat in the microwave before serving.

Nutrition Facts per Serving:

Calories: 311, Fats: 20.4g, Carbs: 32g, Fiber: 5.6g, Sugar: 9.4g, Proteins: 7g, Sodium: 244mg

Banana Curry

Prep time: 15 minutes, Cook time: 15 minutes; Serves 4

Ingredients:

- 2 tablespoons olive oil
- 2 onions, chopped
- 8 garlic cloves, minced
- ½ cup curry powder
- 1 tablespoon ground ginger
- 1 tablespoon ground cumin
- 1 teaspoon ground turmeric
- 1 teaspoon ground cinnamon
- 1 teaspoon red chili powder
- Salt and ground black pepper, as required
- 2/3 cup soy yogurt
- 1 cup tomato puree
- 2 bananas, peeled and sliced
- 3 tomatoes, chopped finely
- ¼ cup unsweetened coconut flakes

Instructions:

1. In a large pan, heat the oil over medium heat and sauté onion for about 4-5 minutes.
2. Add the garlic, curry powder and spices and sauté for about 1 minute.
3. Add the soy yogurt and tomato sauce and bring to a gentle boil.
4. Stir in the bananas and simmer for about 3 minutes.
5. Stir in the tomatoes and simmer for about 1-2 minutes.
6. Stir in the coconut flakes and immediately remove from the heat.
7. Serve hot.

Meal Prep Tip:

1. Transfer the curry into a large bowl and set aside to cool.
2. Divide the mixture into 4 airtight containers.
3. Cover and refrigerate for 2 days.
4. Reheat in the microwave before serving.

Nutrition Facts per Serving:

Calories: 315, Fats: 41.8g, Carbs: 45.3g, Fiber: 11.4g, Sugar: 18.9g, Proteins: 7.7g, Sodium: 315mg

Butternut Squash Curry

Prep time: 15 minutes, Cook time: 35 minutes; Serves 6

Ingredients:

- 1 tablespoon coconut oil
- 2 onions, chopped
- 3 tablespoons curry paste
- 2 pounds butternut squash, peeled and cubed
- 4 cups coconut milk
- Salt and ground black pepper, as required
- ¼ cup fresh basil, chopped

Instructions:

1. In a large skillet, heat the oil over medium heat and sauté the onion for about 5 minutes until tender.
2. Add the curry paste and cook for about 1 minute.
3. Add the butternut squash and stir to combine.
4. Add the coconut milk and salt and bring to a boil.
5. Reduce the heat to medium and cook, covered for about 20-25 minutes or until the desired thickness of sauce.
6. Serve hot with the garnishing of basil.

Meal Prep Tip:

1. Transfer the curry into a large bowl and set aside to cool.
2. Divide the mixture into 6 airtight containers.
3. Cover and refrigerate for 2 days.
4. Reheat in the microwave before serving.

Nutrition Facts per Serving:

Calories: 521, Fats: 45g, Carbs: 32.1g, Fiber: 7.4g, Sugar: 10.2g, Proteins: 6g, Sodium: 59mg

Okra Curry

Prep time: 10 minutes, Cook time: 13 minutes; Serves 2

Ingredients:

- 1 tablespoon olive oil
- ½ teaspoon cumin seeds
- ¾ pound okra pods, trimmed and cut into 2-inch pieces
- ½ teaspoon curry powder
- ½ teaspoon red chili powder
- 1 teaspoon ground coriander
- Salt and ground black pepper, as required

Instructions:

1. In a large skillet, heat the oil over medium heat and sauté the cumin seeds for about 30 seconds.
2. Add the okra and stir fry for about 1-1½ minutes.
3. Reduce the heat to low and simmer, covered for about 6-8 minutes, stirring occasionally.
4. Uncover and increase the heat to medium.
5. Stir in the curry powder, red chili and coriander and cook for about 2-3 minutes more.
6. Season with the salt and remove from the heat.
7. Serve hot.

Meal Prep Tip:

1. Transfer the curry into a large bowl and set aside to cool.
2. Divide the mixture into 2 airtight containers.
3. Cover and refrigerate for 2 days.
4. Reheat in the microwave before serving.

Nutrition Facts per Serving:

Calories: 134, Fats: 7.6g, Carbs: 13.6g, Fiber: 5.9g, Sugar: 2.6g, Proteins: 7.6g, Sodium: 134mg

Spicy Veggies Combo

Prep time: 20 minutes, Cook time: 10 minutes; Serves 5

Ingredients:

- 2 tablespoons vegetable oil
- 2 garlic cloves, minced
- 1 Serrano pepper, chopped
- 1½ cups zucchini, halved lengthwise and sliced
- 1½ cups fresh mushrooms, sliced
- 1 cup fresh broccoli florets
- 1 large red bell pepper, seeded and sliced
- 1 yellow bell pepper, seeded and sliced
- 3 tablespoons soy sauce
- 1 tablespoon balsamic vinegar
- Ground black pepper, as required

Instructions:

1. In a large skillet, heat oil over medium-high heat and sauté the garlic for about 1 minute.
2. Add the zucchini and mushrooms and stir fry for about 2 minutes.
3. Add the broccoli and bell peppers and stir fry for about 2-3 minutes.
4. Stir in the soy sauce and vinegar and stir fry for about 3-4 minutes.
5. Season with the black pepper and remove from the heat.
6. Serve hot.

Meal Prep Tip:

1. Transfer the veggie mixture into a large bowl and set aside to cool.
2. Divide the mixture into 5 airtight containers.
3. Cover and refrigerate for 2 days.
4. Reheat in the microwave before serving.

Nutrition Facts per Serving:

Calories: 87, Fats: 1.9g, Carbs: 7.9g, Fiber: 1.9g, Sugar: 3.9g, Proteins: 2.8g, Sodium: 553mg

Mixed Veggie Noodles

Prep time: 20 minutes, Cook time: 13 minutes; Serves 4

Ingredients:

- 1½ tablespoons sunflower oil
- ¼ cup onion, chopped
- 2 garlic cloves, minced
- 1 jalapeño pepper, seeded and chopped
- 1 large carrot, peeled and spiralized
- 1 large zucchini, spiralized
- 1 large yellow squash, spiralized
- 2 tablespoons fresh lemon juice
- Salt and ground black pepper, as required
- ½ cup scallion, chopped

Instructions:

1. In a large skillet, heat the oil over medium heat and sauté the onion for about 4-5 minutes.
2. Add the garlic and jalapeño pepper and sauté for about 1 minute.
3. Add the carrot noodles and cook for about 2-3 minutes.
4. Add the squash and zucchini noodles and cook for about 3-4 minutes.
5. Stir in the lime juice, salt and black pepper and remove from the heat.
6. Serve immediately with the topping of scallion.

Meal Prep Tip:

1. Transfer the veggie noodles mixture into a large bowl and set aside to cool.
2. Divide the mixture into 4 airtight containers.
3. Cover and refrigerate for 2 days.
4. Reheat in the microwave before serving.

Nutrition Facts per Serving:

Calories: 92, Fats: 5.7g, Carbs: 9.6g, Fiber: 2.9g, Sugar: 4.6g, Proteins: 2.6g, Sodium: 71mg

Tempeh in Tomato Sauce

Prep time: 15 minutes, Cook time: 1 hour 20 minutes; Serves 4

Ingredients:

- ½ cup vegetable oil, divided
- 2 (8-ounce) packages tempeh, cut into ½-inch slices horizontally
- 1 large onion, chopped
- 3 garlic cloves, minced
- 1 teaspoon dried oregano, crushed
- 1 teaspoon dried thyme, crushed
- 1 teaspoon red chili powder
- 1 teaspoon paprika
- 2 large green bell peppers, seeded and sliced thinly
- 4 cups tomatoes, chopped finely
- 1 teaspoon balsamic vinegar
- 1 tablespoon maple syrup

Instructions:

1. Preheat the oven to 350 degrees F.
2. In a large bowl, add 2 tablespoons of the oil and tempeh slices and toss to coat well.
3. In a large skillet, heat ¼ cup of oil over medium-high heat and cook the tempeh slices for about 5-7 minutes per side.
4. Transfer the cooked tempeh slices into a paper towel-lined plate. Set aside.
5. Meanwhile, in another nonstick skillet, heat the remaining oil over medium-low heat and sauté the onion, garlic, herbs and spices for about 8-10 minutes.
6. Add the bell pepper and sauté for about 10 minutes.
7. Add the remaining ingredients and stir until well combined.
8. Transfer the tempeh slices into a large casserole dish.
9. Place the tomato mixture over tempeh slices evenly.
10. With a foil paper, cover the casserole dish and bake for about 1 hour.
11. Remove from the oven and serve hot.

Meal Prep Tip:

1. Transfer the tempeh mixture into a large bowl and set aside to cool.
2. Divide the mixture into 4 airtight containers.
3. Cover and refrigerate for 2 days.
4. Reheat in the microwave before serving.

Nutrition Facts per Serving:

Calories: 548, Fats: 40.3g, Carbs: 30.8g, Fiber: 4.5g, Sugar: 12.5g, Proteins: 24g, Sodium: 30mg

Tofu with Peas

Prep time: 15 minutes, Cook time: 15 minutes; Serves 6

Ingredients:

- 1 tablespoon chile garlic sauce
- 3 tablespoons soy sauce
- 2 tablespoons canola oil, divided
- 1 (16-ounce) package extra-firm tofu, drained, pressed and cubed
- 1 cup onion, chopped
- 1 tablespoon fresh ginger, minced
- 2 garlic cloves, minced
- 1 cup frozen peas, thawed
- 2½ cups snow peas, trimmed
- 2½ cups sugar snap peas, trimmed
- 1 teaspoon sesame seeds

Instructions:

1. For sauce: in a bowl, add the chile garlic sauce and soy sauce and mix until well combined.
2. In a large skillet, heat 1 tablespoon of the oil over medium-high heat and cook the tofu for about 4-5 minutes or until browned completely, stirring occasionally.
3. Transfer the tofu into a bowl
4. In the same skillet, heat the remaining oil over medium heat and sauté the onion for about 3-4 minutes.
5. Add the ginger and garlic and sauté for about 1 minute.
6. Stir in all three peas and cook for about 2-3 minutes.
7. Stir in the sauce mixture and tofu and cook for about 1-2 minutes.
8. Serve hot with the garnishing of sesame seeds.

Meal Prep Tip:

1. Transfer the tofu mixture into a large bowl and set aside to cool.
2. Divide the mixture into 6 airtight containers.
3. Cover and refrigerate for 2 days.
4. Reheat in the microwave before serving.

Nutrition Facts per Serving:

Calories: 225, Fats: 7.2g, Carbs: 21.9g, Fiber: 7.2g, Sugar: 9.7g, Proteins: 15.1g, Sodium: 548mg

Chapter 7 Salad Recipes

Mixed Veggie Salad

Prep time: 25 minutes, Serves 8

Ingredients:

For Dressing:

- 1/3 cup olive oil
- ½ cup fresh lemon juice
- 1 tablespoon fresh ginger, grated
- 2 teaspoons whole grain mustard
- 2 teaspoons maple syrup
- ¼ teaspoon salt

For Salad:

- 2 avocados, peeled, pitted and chopped
- 2 tablespoons fresh lemon juice
- 2 cups fresh baby kale, sliced thinly
- 2 cups small broccoli florets
- 1 cup red cabbage, shredded
- 1 cup purple cabbage, shredded
- 2 large carrots, peeled and grated
- 1 small orange bell pepper, seeded and sliced into matchsticks
- 1 small yellow bell pepper, seeded and sliced into matchsticks
- ½ cup fresh parsley leaves, chopped
- 1 cup walnuts, chopped

Instructions:

1. For dressing: in a food processor, add all the ingredients and pulse until well combined and smooth.
2. For salad: in a bowl, add the avocado slices and lime juice and toss to coat well.
3. Add the remaining vegetables and toss to coat well.
4. Top with walnuts and serve immediately.

Meal Prep Tip:

1. Transfer dressing into a small jar and refrigerate for 1 day.
2. In 8 containers, divide avocado and remaining vegetables.
3. Cover the containers and refrigerate for 1 day.
4. Before serving, drizzle each portion with dressing and serve with the topping of walnuts

Nutrition Facts per Serving:

Calories: 321, Fats: 27.8g, Carbs: 16.4g, Fiber: 6.8g, Sugar: 5.1g, Proteins: 6.8g, Sodium: 119mg

Tofu & Veggies Salad

Prep time: 20 minutes; Serves 5

Ingredients:

For Dressing:

- ½ cup smooth peanut butter
- ¼ cup balsamic vinegar
- 3 tablespoons soy sauce
- 2 tablespoons water
- 1 teaspoon sesame oil, toasted
- 1 teaspoon Sriracha

For Salad:

- 6 ounces broccoli, chopped
- 6 ounces cabbage, shredded
- 1 small red bell pepper, seeded and julienned
- 1 small yellow bell pepper, seeded and julienned
- 1 pound baked tofu, cubed
- ¼ cup edamame, shelled and cooked
- ¼ cup peanuts, roasted
- ¼ cup fresh cilantro leaves

Instructions:

1. For dressing: in a bowl, add all the ingredients and beat until well combined.
2. For salad: in a large bowl, add all the ingredients and mix well.
3. Place the dressing over the salad and toss to coat well.
4. Serve immediately.

Meal Prep Tip:

1. Transfer the dressing into a container and refrigerate for 1 day.
2. In a large container, mix together broccoli, cabbage and bell peppers. Cover and refrigerate for 1 day.
3. Before serving, divide salad onto serving plates.
4. Top with the tofu, edamame, peanuts, and cilantro.
5. Drizzle with dressing and serve.

Nutrition Facts per Serving:

Calories: 327, Fats: 22.4g, Carbs: 18.1g, Fiber: 6g, Sugar: 7.5g, Proteins: 29.9g, Sodium: 700mg

Farro & Zucchini Salad

Prep time: 15 minutes, Serves 3

Ingredients:

- 6 teaspoons extra-virgin olive oil
- 2 teaspoons balsamic vinegar
- Salt and ground black pepper, as required
- 2 medium zucchinis, spiralized with Blade C
- 2 cups cooked farro
- 2½ cups grape tomatoes
- ¼ cup fresh basil leaves

Instructions:

1. In a small bowl, add oil, vinegar, salt and black pepper and beat until well combined.
2. In a large bowl, add the remaining ingredients and mix well.
3. Pour the vinaigrette over salad and toss to coat well.
4. Serve immediately.

Instructions:

1. In the bottom of 3 large mason jars, divide the vinaigrette.
2. Divide the salad ingredients in the layers of zucchini, farro, tomatoes and basil.
3. Cover each jar with the lid tightly and refrigerate for about 1 day.
4. Shake the jars well just before serving.

Nutrition Facts per Serving:

Calories: 556, Fats: 9.9g, Carbs: 98.3g, Fiber: 111.3g, Sugar: 6.2g, Proteins: 21.6g, Sodium: 151mg

Chickpeas & Veggie Salad

Prep time: 15 minutes, Serves 4

Ingredients:

For Dressing:

- 1 garlic clove, minced
- 1/3 cup extra-virgin olive oil
- 2 tablespoons fresh lemon juice
- 1 teaspoon balsamic vinegar
- ¼ teaspoon dried oregano
- ¼ teaspoon dried parsley
- Salt and freshly ground black pepper, to taste

For Salad:

- 1 small cucumber, peeled, seeded and cubed
- 1/3 cup Kalamata olives, pitted and halved
- 1 (15¼-ounce) can chickpeas, rinsed, drained and patted dry
- 1 small onion, sliced thinly
- 1 cup grape tomatoes, halved
- 3 tablespoons pine nuts
- 5 cups romaine lettuce, torn
- 2 cups fresh baby spinach, torn

Instructions:

1. For dressing: in a bowl, add all the ingredients and beat until well combined.
2. For salad: in a large bowl, add all the ingredients and mix well.
3. Place the dressing over the salad and toss to coat well.
4. Serve immediately.

Meal Prep Tip:

1. In the bottom of 4 mason jars, divide the dressing.
2. Add the salad ingredients in the layers of cucumber, followed by olives, chickpeas, onion, tomatoes, pine nuts, lettuce and spinach.
3. Cover each jar with the lid tightly and refrigerate for about 1 day.
4. Shake the jars well just before serving.

Nutrition Facts per Serving:

Calories: 359, Fats: 23.7g, Carbs: 29.4g, Fiber: 7.2g, Sugar: 4.3g, Proteins: 9.2g, Sodium: 185mg

Chickpeas & Quinoa Salad

Prep time: 15 minutes, Serves 4

Ingredients:

For Dressing:

- 2 tablespoons olive oil
- 2 tablespoons fresh lemon juice
- ¼ teaspoon dried oregano
- Salt and ground black pepper, as required

For Salad:

- 6 cups fresh kale, trimmed and chopped
- 1 cup cooked quinoa
- 1 cup tomato, chopped
- 1 cup cucumber, chopped
- ½ cup chickpeas
- ½ cup Kalamata olives
- 4 tablespoons hummus
- 2 tablespoons fresh dill, chopped
- 1 lemon, quartered

Instructions:

1. For dressing: in a bowl, add all the ingredients and beat until well combined.
2. For salad: in a large bowl, add all the ingredients and mix well.
3. Place the dressing over the salad and toss to coat well.
4. Serve immediately.

Instructions:

1. In the bottom of 4 mason jars, divide the dressing.
2. Add the salad ingredients in the layers of quinoa, kale, tomatoes, cucumber, chickpeas, feta olives, hummus, dill and lemon.
3. Cover each jar with the lid tightly and refrigerate for about 1 day.
4. Shake the jars well just before serving.

Nutrition Facts per Serving:

Calories: 354, Fats: 13.5g, Carbs: 49.1g, Fiber: 8.3g, Sugar: 2g, Proteins: 12.7g, Sodium: 335mg

Quinoa & Veggies Salad

Prep time: 20 minutes, Cook time: 16 minutes; Serves 4

Ingredients:

For Quinoa:

- 1 teaspoon olive oil
- 1 cup golden quinoa, rinsed and drained
- 1¾ cups homemade vegetable broth

For Salad:

- 1 large seedless cucumber, chopped
- 8 small radishes, trimmed and chopped
- 1 large shallot, chopped
- ½ cup dates, pitted and chopped
- ½ cup almonds, chopped

For Vinaigrette:

- 1 tablespoon fresh dill, minced
- 1 teaspoon lemon zest, grated finely
- 3 tablespoons extra-virgin olive oil
- 2 tablespoons fresh lemon juice
- ½ tablespoon balsamic vinegar
- Salt and ground black pepper, as required

Instructions:

1. For quinoa: in a pan, heat oil over medium-high heat and cook the quinoa for about 1 minute, stirring continuously.
2. Add the broth and bring to a boil.
3. Reduce the heat to low and simmer, covered for about 15 minutes or until all the liquid is absorbed.
4. Remove from the heat and set aside, covered for about 5 minutes.
5. Uncover and with a fork, fluff the quinoa.
6. Set aside to cool completely.
7. In a large bowl, mix together the quinoa and all salad ingredients.
8. For vinaigrette: in another bowl, add all the ingredients and beat until well combined.
9. Pour the vinaigrette over salad and gently, toss to coat well.
10. Serve immediately.

Meal Prep Tip:

1. In the bottom of 4 large mason jars, place the vinaigrette evenly.
2. Add the salad ingredients in the layers of quinoa, cucumber, radishes, shallot and dates.
3. Cover each jar with the lid tightly and refrigerate for about 1 day.
4. Shake the jars well just before serving.
5. Top with almonds and serve.

Nutrition Facts per Serving:

Calories: 336, Fats: 13.4g, Carbs: 49.8g, Fiber: 5.9g, Sugar: 16.6g, Proteins: 7.4g, Sodium: 282mg

Beans & Couscous Salad

Prep time: 20 minutes, Cook time: 5 minutes; Serves 6

Ingredients:

For Salad:

- ½ cup homemade vegetable broth
- ½ cup couscous
- 1 cup cucumber, chopped
- 2 cups canned garbanzo beans, rinsed and drained
- 1 cup plum tomato, chopped
- 1½ cups canned cannellini beans, rinsed and drained
- 1½ cups canned black beans, rinsed and drained

For Dressing:

- 1 garlic clove, minced
- 2 tablespoons shallots, minced
- 2 teaspoons lemon zest, grated finely
- ¼ cup fresh lemon juice
- 2 tablespoons extra-virgin olive oil
- Salt and ground black pepper, as required

Instructions:

1. In a pan, add the broth over medium heat and bring to a boil.
2. Add the couscous and stir to combine.
3. Cover the pan and immediately remove from the heat.
4. Set aside for about 5-10 minutes or until all the liquid is absorbed.
5. For salad: in a large serving bowl, add the couscous and remaining ingredients and stir to combine.
6. For dressing: in another small bowl, add all the ingredients and beat until well combined.
7. Pour the dressing over salad and gently, toss to coat well.
8. Serve immediately.

Meal Prep Tip:

1. In the bottom of 6 large mason jars, divide the dressing evenly.
2. Divide the salad ingredients in the layers of cucumber, followed by the garbanzo beans, tomato cannellini beans, black beans and couscous.
3. Cover each jar with the lid tightly and refrigerate for about 1 day.
4. Shake the jars well just before serving.

Nutrition Facts per Serving:

Calories: 414, Fats: 6.4g, Carbs: 67.4g, Fiber: 16.9g, Sugar: 2.4g, Proteins: 22g, Sodium: 126mg

Chickpeas & Lentil Salad

Prep time: 15 minutes, Cook time: 35 minutes; Serves 5

Ingredients:

- 1½ cups water
- ½ cup dry lentils
- 1 (15-ounce) can chickpeas, rinsed and drained
- 1 green bell pepper, seeded and chopped
- 1 yellow bell pepper, seeded and chopped
- 1 red bell pepper, seeded and chopped
- 2 tomatoes, chopped
- 4 scallions, chopped
- 2 jalapeño peppers, minced
- 2 tablespoon olive oil
- 2 tablespoons fresh lime juice
- Salt, as required
- ¼ cup fresh cilantro, chopped

Instructions:

1. In a large pan, add the water and lentils over high heat and bring to a boil.
2. Reduce the heat to low and simmer, covered for about 30 minutes or until all the liquid is absorbed and lentils become tender.
3. Transfer the lentils into a large bowl and set aside to cool completely.
4. After cooling, add the remaining all ingredients and toss to coat well.
5. Serve immediately.

Meal Prep Tip:

1. In 5 containers, divide salad evenly.
2. Cover the container and refrigerate for about 1 day.
3. Shake well before serving.

Nutrition Facts per Serving:

Calories: 226, Fats: 7.2g, Carbs: 31.8g, Fiber: 10.4g, Sugar: 6.1g, Proteins: 10.2g, Sodium: 318mg

Mixed Grains Salad

Prep time: 20 minutes, Serves 6

Ingredients:

For Dressing:

- ¼ cup fresh lime juice
- 2 tablespoons maple syrup
- 1 tablespoon Dijon mustard
- 1 teaspoon white sugar
- ½ teaspoon ground cumin
- 1 teaspoon garlic powder
- Salt and ground black pepper, as required
- ½ cup extra-virgin olive oil

For Salad:

- 2 cups fresh mango, peeled, pitted and cubed
- 2 tablespoon fresh lime juice, divided
- 2 avocados, peeled, pitted and cubed
- Pinch of salt
- 1 cup cooked quinoa
- 2 (14-ounce) cans black beans, rinsed and drained
- 1 (15¼-ounce) can corn, rinsed and drained
- 1 small onion, chopped
- 1 jalapeño, seeded and chopped finely
- ½ cup fresh cilantro, chopped
- 6 cups romaine lettuce, shredded

Instructions:

1. For dressing: in a blender, add all the ingredients except oil and pulse until well combined.
2. While the motor is running, slowly add oil and pulse until smooth.
3. For salad: in a bowl, add the mango and 1 tablespoon of lime juice and toss to coat well.
4. In another bowl, add the avocado, a pinch of salt and remaining lime juice and toss to coat well.
5. In a large serving bowl, add the mango, avocado and remaining salad ingredients and mix.
6. Place the dressing and toss to coat well.
7. Serve immediately.

Meal Prep Tip:

1. In the bottom of 6 large mason jars, divide the dressing evenly.
2. Divide the salad ingredients in the layers of quinoa, followed by mango, black beans, corns, avocado, onion, jalapeño, cilantro and lettuce.
3. Cover each jar with the lid tightly and refrigerate for about 1 day.
4. Shake the jars well just before serving.

Nutrition Facts per Serving:

Calories: 612, Fats: 31.6g, Carbs: 73g, Fiber: 15.7g, Sugar: 15.8g, Proteins: 15.7g, Sodium: 260mg

Beans & Corn Salad

Prep time: 15 minutes; Serves 8

Ingredients:

For Salad:

- 1 (10-ounce) package frozen corn kernels, thawed
- 1 (15-ounce) can black beans, rinsed and drained
- 1 (15-ounce) can kidney beans, rinsed and drained
- 1 (15-ounce) can cannellini beans, rinsed and drained
- 2 large bell peppers, seeded and chopped
- 1 large red onion, chopped

For Dressing:

- ¼ cup fresh cilantro, minced
- 1 garlic clove, minced
- 1 tablespoon maple syrup
- ½ cup balsamic vinegar
- ½ cup olive oil
- 1 tablespoon fresh lime juice
- 1 tablespoon fresh lemon juice
- Drop of hot sauce
- ½ teaspoon red pepper flakes, crushed
- Salt and ground black pepper, as required

Instructions:

1. For salad: add all the ingredients in a large serving bowl and mix well.
2. For dressing: add all the ingredients in a bowl and beat until well combined.
3. Place the dressing over salad and gently toss to coat well.
4. Serve immediately.

Meal Prep Tip:

1. Divide salad into 8 airtight containers.
2. Cover the containers and refrigerate for 1-2 days.
3. Shake well before serving.

Nutrition Facts per Serving:

Calories: 298, Fats: 11.5g, Carbs: 37.7g, Fiber: 11.5g, Sugar: 6.2g, Proteins: 10.9g, Sodium: 143mg

Corn & Veggie Salad

Prep time: 15 minutes, Serves 4

Ingredients:

For Salad:

- 4 cups frozen corn kernels, thawed
- 1 small green bell pepper, seeded and chopped
- 1 small orange bell pepper, seeded and chopped
- 1 small red bell pepper, seeded and chopped
- 2 tomatoes, chopped
- 1 red onion, chopped
- 2 tablespoons fresh mint leaves

For Dressing:

- 2 tablespoons fresh cilantro, minced
- 1 garlic clove, minced
- 2 tablespoons extra-virgin olive oil
- 2 tablespoons fresh lemon juice
- Salt and ground black pepper, as required

Instructions:

1. For salad: add all the ingredients except mint in a large serving bowl and mix well.
2. For dressing: add all the ingredients in a bowl and beat until well combined.
3. Place the dressing over salad and gently toss to coat well.
4. Serve with the garnishing of mint.

Meal Prep Tip:

1. Divide salad into 8 airtight containers.
2. Cover the containers and refrigerate for 1-2 days.
3. Shake well before serving.

Nutrition Facts per Serving:

Calories: 248, Fats: 8.6g, Carbs: 44g, Fiber: 6.7g, Sugar: 12.5g, Proteins: 6.1g, Sodium: 50mg

Black Beans & Mango Salad

Prep time: 15 minutes, Serves 6

Ingredients:

For Salad:

- 2 (15½-ounce) cans black beans, rinsed and drained
- 2 mangoes, peeled, pitted and chopped
- ½ cup red onion, chopped
- 2 tablespoons fresh cilantro, chopped

For Dressing:

- 1 (½-inch) pieces fresh ginger, grated
- 2 teaspoons fresh orange zest, grated finely
- 3-4 tablespoons fresh orange juice
- 1 tablespoon apple cider vinegar
- 2 teaspoons extra-virgin olive oil
- ¼ teaspoon red pepper flakes, crushed
- Salt, as required

Instructions:

1. For salad: add all the ingredients in a large serving bowl and mix well.
2. For dressing: add all the ingredients in a bowl and beat until well combined.
3. Place the dressing over salad and gently toss to coat well.
4. Serve immediately.

Meal Prep Tip:

1. Divide salad into 6 airtight containers.
2. Cover the containers and refrigerate for 1-2 days.
3. Shake well before serving.

Nutrition Facts per Serving:

Calories: 222, Fats: 3.2g, Carbs: 40.4g, Fiber: 9.3g, Sugar: 16.4g, Proteins: 9.6g, Sodium: 47mg

Kidney Beans & Pomegranate Salad

Prep time: 15 minutes, Serves 3

Ingredients:

- 2 cups canned white kidney beans, rinsed and drained
- 1 cup fresh pomegranate seeds
- 1/3 cup scallion (green part), chopped finely
- 2 tablespoons fresh parsley, chopped
- 1 tablespoon fresh lime juice
- Salt and ground black pepper, as required

Instructions:

1. In a large serving bowl, place all the ingredients and toss to coat well.
2. Serve immediately.

Meal Prep Tip:

1. Divide salad into 3 airtight containers.
2. Cover the containers and refrigerate for 1-2 days.
3. Shake well before serving.

Nutrition Facts per Serving:

Calories: 180, Fats: 0g, Carbs: 34.9g, Fiber: 14.1g, Sugar: 5.3g, Proteins: 11.4g, Sodium: 74mg

Rice & Tofu Salad

Prep time: 15 minutes, Serves 4

Ingredients:

For Salad:

- 1 (12-ounce) package tofu, drained and sliced
- 1½ cups cooked brown rice
- ½ of cucumber, peeled, seeded and chopped
- ½ of head romaine lettuce, torn

For Dressing:

- 3 scallions, chopped
- 2 tablespoons black sesame seeds, toasted
- 2 tablespoons soy sauce
- ½ teaspoon sesame oil, toasted
- Drop of hot pepper sauce
- 1 tablespoon maple syrup
- ¼ teaspoon chile pepper powder

Instructions:

1. In a large serving bowl, place all the ingredients and toss to coat well.
2. Serve immediately.

Meal Prep Tip:

1. Divide salad into 4 airtight containers.
2. Cover the containers and refrigerate for 1-2 days.
3. Shake well before serving.

Nutrition Facts per Serving:

Calories: 380, Fats: 8.4g, Carbs: 64.2g, Fiber: 4.5g, Sugar: 4.9g, Proteins: 14.2g, Sodium: 470mg

Chapter 8 Snacks And Sides Recipes

Steamed Green Beans

Prep time: 10 minutes, Cook time: 8 minutes; Serves 5

Ingredients:

- 1½ pounds fresh green beans, trimmed
- 1 tablespoon olive oil
- Salt and ground black pepper, as required

Instructions:

1. In a large pan of boiling water, arrange steamer basket.
2. Place green beans in steamer basket.
3. Cover and steam for about 7-8 minutes or until desired doneness.
4. Drain well and transfer the beans into a bowl.
5. Drizzle with oil and sprinkle with salt and black pepper and toss to coat.
6. Serve immediately.

Meal Prep Tip:

1. Transfer the green beans into a large bowl and set aside to cool.
2. Divide the green beans into 5 airtight containers.
3. Cover and refrigerate for 2 days.
4. Reheat in the microwave before serving.

Nutrition Facts per Serving:

Calories: 66, Fats: 0.4g, Carbs: 9.7g, Fiber: 4.6g, Sugar: 1.9g, Proteins: 2.5g, Sodium: 39mg

Stir Fried Asparagus

Prep time: 10 minutes, Cook time: 5 minutes; Serves 5

Ingredients:

- 1 tablespoon vegetable oil
- 1½ pounds asparagus, trimmed and cut into 2-inch pieces
- Salt and ground black pepper, as required
- 3 garlic cloves, minced
- 1 tablespoon fresh ginger, grated
- 1 Serrano pepper, chopped finely

Instructions:

1. In a large skillet, heat the oil over medium-high heat and stir fry the asparagus with salt and black pepper for about 2 minutes.
2. Add the garlic, ginger and Serrano pepper and stir-fry for about 2-3 minutes.
3. Serve hot.

Meal Prep Tip:

1. Transfer the green beans into a large bowl and set aside to cool.
2. Divide the green beans into 5 airtight containers.
3. Cover and refrigerate for 2 days.
4. Reheat in the microwave before serving.

Nutrition Facts per Serving:

Calories: 58, Fats: 3g, Carbs: 6.7g, Fiber: 3.1g, Sugar: 2.7g, Proteins: 3.2g, Sodium: 35mg

Roasted Brussels Sprout

Prep time: 15 minutes, Cook time: 50 minutes; Serves 6

Ingredients:

- 2 pounds small-sized Brussels sprouts, trimmed
- 1 tablespoon fresh rosemary, minced
- Salt and ground black pepper, as required
- 1 tablespoon olive oil

Instructions:

1. Preheat the oven to 425 degrees F. Grease 2 large shallow roasting pans.
2. In a roasting pan, place Brussels sprouts.
3. Sprinkle with rosemary, salt and black pepper and drizzle with oil.
4. Roast for about 45-50 minutes.
5. Remove from the oven and serve hot.

Meal Prep Tip:

1. Transfer the Brussels sprouts into a large bowl and set aside to cool.
2. Divide the Brussels sprouts into 6 airtight containers.
3. Cover and refrigerate for 2 days.
4. Reheat in the microwave before serving.

Nutrition Facts per Serving:

Calories: 87, Fats: 2.9g, Carbs: 14.1g, Fiber: 5.9g, Sugar: 3.3g, Proteins: 5.2g, Sodium: 65mg

Stir Fried Broccoli

Prep time: 10 minutes, Cook time: 8 minutes; Serves 2

Ingredients:

- 1 tablespoon olive oil
- 1 garlic clove, minced
- 1 fresh red chili, seeded and chopped
- 2 cups broccoli florets
- 2 tablespoons soy sauce

Instructions:

1. In a large skillet, heat the oil over medium heat and sauté the garlic and red chili for about 1 minute.
2. Add the broccoli and stir fry for about 2 minutes.
3. Stir in the soy sauce and stir fry for about 4-5 minutes.
4. Serve warm.

Meal Prep Tip:

1. Transfer the broccoli into a large bowl and set aside to cool.
2. Divide the broccoli into 2 airtight containers.
3. Cover and refrigerate for 2 days.
4. Reheat in the microwave before serving.

Nutrition Facts per Serving:

Calories: 103, Fats: 7.3g, Carbs: 8g, Fiber: 2.6g, Sugar: 2g, Proteins: 3.7g, Sodium: 933mg

Sautéed Zucchini

Prep time: 15 minutes, Cook time: 14 minutes; Serves 8

Ingredients:

- 3 tablespoons olive oil
- 1 jalapeño pepper, seeded and minced
- 2 garlic cloves, minced
- 2 pounds zucchini, sliced diagonally
- 1 teaspoon Italian seasoning
- Salt and ground black pepper, as required

Instructions:

1. In a large skillet, heat the oil over medium heat and sauté the jalapeño pepper and garlic for about 1 minute.
2. Add the zucchini and cook for about 5-6 minutes.
3. Stir in the Italian seasoning, salt and black pepper and cook for about 1 minute.
4. Serve hot.

Meal Prep Tip:

1. Transfer the zucchini into a large bowl and set aside to cool.
2. Divide the zucchini into 8 airtight containers.
3. Cover and refrigerate for 2 days.
4. Reheat in the microwave before serving.

Nutrition Facts per Serving:

Calories: 67, Fats: 5.6g, Carbs: 4.2g, Fiber: 1.3g, Sugar: 2.1g, Proteins: 1.4g, Sodium: 31mg

Soy Sauce Zucchini Noodles

Prep time: 15 minutes, Cook time: 2 minutes; Serves 2

Ingredients:

- ½ tablespoon extra-virgin olive oil, divided
- 1 large zucchini, spiralized with Blade C
- Ground black pepper, as required
- 1 tablespoon low-sodium soy sauce
- 1 tablespoon fresh parsley, chopped

Instructions:

1. In a microwave-safe bowl, place the zucchini noodles.
2. Sprinkle with salt and black pepper and microwave on High for about 1 minute.
3. Drizzle with the oil and soy sauce and microwave for about 1 minute more.
4. Transfer zucchini in a large serving plate and serve with the garnishing of parsley.

Meal Prep Tip:

1. Transfer the zucchini noodles into a large bowl and set aside to cool.
2. Divide the zucchini noodles into 2 airtight containers.
3. Cover and refrigerate for 2 days.
4. Reheat in the microwave before serving.

Nutrition Facts per Serving:

Calories: 59, Fats: 3.8g, Carbs: 6.1g, Fiber: 1.9g, Sugar: 3.3g, Proteins: 2.5g, Sodium: 457mg

Spiced Corn

Prep time: 10 minutes, Cook time: 10 minutes; Serves 4

Ingredients:

- 1 tablespoon olive oil
- 1 (16-ounce) package frozen corn
- 1 plum tomato, chopped
- 1 tablespoon fresh lime juice
- Salt, as required
- ½ teaspoon ground cumin
- 1/3 cup fresh cilantro, minced

Instructions:

1. In a large cast iron skillet, melt the butter over medium-high heat and cook the corn for about 3-5 minutes, stirring occasionally.
2. Add the tomato, lime juice, cumin and salt and stir to combine.
3. Reduce the heat to medium-low and cook for about 3-4 minutes.
4. Stir in the cilantro and remove from the heat.
5. Serve hot.

Meal Prep Tip:

1. Transfer the corn mixture into a large bowl and set aside to cool.
2. Divide the mixture into 5 airtight containers.
3. Cover and refrigerate for 2 days.
4. Reheat in the microwave before serving.

Nutrition Facts per Serving:

Calories: 120, Fats: 4.2g, Carbs: 25.2g, Fiber: 3.9g, Sugar: 2.9g, Proteins: 3.9g, Sodium: 95mg

Basil Cauliflower

Prep time: 15 minutes, Cook time: 8 minutes; Serves 4

Ingredients:

- ½ cup homemade vegetable broth
- 4 cups fresh cauliflower florets
- 2 shallots, chopped
- 1 teaspoon dried basil, crushed
- ½ teaspoon seasoned salt
- Ground black pepper, as required

Instructions:

1. In a large cast iron skillet, add all the ingredients and mix well.
2. Place the skillet over medium heat and cook for about 6-8 minutes, stirring occasionally.
3. Serve hot.

Meal Prep Tip:

1. Transfer the cauliflower mixture into a large bowl and set aside to cool.
2. Divide the cauliflower mixture into 4 airtight containers.
3. Cover and refrigerate for 2 days.
4. Reheat in the microwave before serving.

Nutrition Facts per Serving:

Calories: 36, Fats: 0.3g, Carbs: 7g, Fiber: 2.5g, Sugar: 2.5g, Proteins: 2.8g, Sodium: 317mg

Sweet & Sour Kale

Prep time: 10 minutes, Cook time: 20 minutes; Serves 4

Ingredients:

- 1 tablespoon extra-virgin olive oil
- 1 lemon, seeded and sliced thinly
- 1 onion, chopped
- 3 garlic cloves, minced
- 2 pound fresh kale, trimmed and chopped
- ½ cup scallions, chopped
- 1 tablespoon maple syrup
- Salt and ground black pepper, as required

Instructions:

1. In a large cast iron skillet, heat the oil over medium heat and cook the lemon slices for about 5 minutes.
2. With a slotted spoon, remove the lemon slices from skillet and set aside.
3. In the same skillet, add the onion and garlic and sauté for about 5 minutes.
4. Add the kale, scallions, honey, salt and pepper and cook for 8-10 minutes.
5. Add the lemon slices and mix until well combined.
6. Serve hot.

Meal Prep Tip:

1. Transfer the kale mixture into a large bowl and set aside to cool.
2. Divide the kale mixture into 4 airtight containers.
3. Cover and refrigerate for 2 days.
4. Reheat in the microwave before serving.

Nutrition Facts per Serving:

Calories: 174, Fats: 3.6g, Carbs: 31.6g, Fiber: 4.5g, Sugar: 4.6g, Proteins: 7.5g, Sodium: 141mg

Nutty Spinach

Prep time: 10 minutes, Cook time: 5 minutes; Serves 2

Ingredients:

- 1 tablespoon olive oil
- 6 cups fresh spinach
- 2 garlic cloves, chopped finely
- Salt, as required
- 2 tablespoons almonds, sliced

Instructions:

1. In a large skillet, heat the oil over medium-high heat and cook the spinach for about 1 minute, stirring continuously.
2. Add the garlic and salt and cook or about 2-3 minutes or until wilted.
3. Stir in almond slices and remove from the heat.
4. Serve hot.

Meal Prep Tip:

1. Transfer the spinach mixture into a large bowl and set aside to cool.
2. Divide the spinach mixture into 2 airtight containers.
3. Cover and refrigerate for 2 days.
4. Reheat in the microwave before serving.

Nutrition Facts per Serving:

Calories: 120, Fats: 10.3g, Carbs: 5.5g, Fiber: 2.8g, Sugar: 0.7g, Proteins: 4g, Sodium: 149mg

Garlicky Mushrooms

Prep time: 10 minutes, Cook time: 8 minutes; Serves 2

Ingredients:

- ½ tablespoon olive oil
- ½ pound fresh button mushrooms, sliced thinly
- 1 teaspoon fresh ginger root, minced
- 1 teaspoon garlic, minced
- 1 tablespoon soy sauce
- Ground black pepper, as required
- 1 tablespoon scallion (green part), chopped

Instructions:

1. In a large skillet, heat the oil over high heat and stir fry the mushrooms for about 5-6 minutes.
2. Add the remaining ingredients except the scallion and stir fry for about 1-2 minutes.
3. Serve hot with the garnishing pf scallion.

Meal Prep Tip:

1. Transfer the mushroom mixture into a large bowl and set aside to cool.
2. Divide the mushroom mixture into 2 airtight containers.
3. Cover and refrigerate for 2 days.
4. Reheat in the microwave before serving.

Nutrition Facts per Serving:

Calories: 62, Fats: 3.9g, Carbs: 5.2g, Fiber: 1.3g, Sugar: 2.2g, Proteins: 4.2g, Sodium: 458mg

Chapter 9 Dessert Recipes

Chocolate Cupcakes

Prep time: 15 minutes, Cook time: 20 minutes; Serves 6

Ingredients:

- 1 cup water
- 1 cup dates, pitted
- 1 cup oat flour
- 1/3 cup unsweetened cocoa powder
- 1 tablespoon baking powder
- ¼ teaspoon salt
- ¼ cup almond milk

Instructions:

1. Preheat oven to 350 degrees F. Line 6 cups of a muffin tin with paper liners.
2. In a food processor, add the water and dates and pulse until smooth.
3. In a large bowl, mix together flour, cacao powder, baking powder and salt.
4. Add the almond milk and date paste and beat until well combined.
5. Transfer the mixture into paper muffin cups about ¾ of full.
6. Bake for 25 minutes or until a toothpick inserted in the center comes out clean.
7. Remove the muffin tin from oven and place onto a wire rack to cool for about 10 minutes.
8. Carefully invert the cupcakes onto the wire rack to cool completely before serving.

Meal Prep Tip:

1. Line an airtight containers with paper towels.
2. Arrange the cooled cupcakes over paper towel in a single layer.
3. Cover the cupcakes with another paper towel.
4. Refrigerate for about 2-3 days.

Nutrition Facts per Serving:

Calories: 180, Fats: 4.2g, Carbs: 37.1g, Fiber: 5.7g, Sugar: 19.2g, Proteins: 3.9g, Sodium: 180mg

Fruity Oat Bars

Prep time: 15 minutes, Cook time: 25 minutes; Serves 6

Ingredients:

- ½ cup rolled oats
- 2 tablespoons flax seeds
- 1 tablespoon sunflower seeds
- 1 tablespoon walnuts, chopped
- 2 tablespoons raisins
- ¾ cup fresh blueberries
- 1 banana, peeled and mashed
- 2 tablespoons dates, pitted and chopped finely
- 1 tablespoon fresh pomegranate juice

Instructions:

1. Preheat the oven to 350 degrees F. Lightly, grease an 8-inch baking dish.
2. In a large bowl, add all ingredients and mix until well combined.
3. Place the mixture into prepared baking dish evenly.
4. Bake for about 25 minutes.
5. Remove from oven and let it cool.
6. With a sharp knife, cut into desired size bars and serve.

Meal Prep Tip:

1. Wrap these bars in wax paper and place into an airtight container.
2. Preserve in refrigerator up to 2 weeks.

Nutrition Facts per Serving:

Calories: 123, Fats: 2.3g, Carbs: 24.5g, Fiber: 2.8g, Sugar: 14.1g, Proteins: 2.3g, Sodium: 5mg

Chickpeas Fudge

Prep time: 15 minutes, Serves 12

Ingredients:

- 2 cups cooked chickpeas
- 8 Medjool dates, pitted and chopped
- ½ cup almond butter
- ½ cup unsweetened almond milk
- 1 teaspoon vanilla extract
- 2 tablespoons unsweetened cocoa powder

Instructions:

1. Line a large baking dish with parchment paper.
2. In a food processor, add all the ingredients except cocoa powder and pulse until well combined.
3. Transfer the mixture into a large bowl and stir in the cocoa powder.
4. Transfer the mixture into the prepared baking dish evenly and with the back of a spatula, smooth the top surface.
5. Refrigerate for about 2 hours or until set completely.
6. Cut into desired sized squares and serve.

Meal Prep Tip:

1. Wrap these squares in wax paper and place into an airtight container.
2. Preserve in refrigerator up to 2 weeks.

Nutrition Facts per Serving:

Calories: 86, Fats: 1.2g, Carbs: 17.5g, Fiber: 2.8g, Sugar: 9.7g, Proteins: 2.6g, Sodium: 73mg

Oat Bars

Prep time: 15 minutes; Serves 12

Ingredients:

- 1½ cups rolled oats
- ½ cup almonds, chopped roughly
- ½ cup cashews, chopped roughly
- ½ cup mini 70% dark chocolate chips
- 1/3 cup pumpkin seeds
- ¼ cup sesame seeds
- ¼ cup sunflower seeds
- ¼ cup flaxseed meal
- 2 tablespoons chia seeds
- 1 teaspoon ground cinnamon
- ½ cup maple syrup
- 1 cup almond butter, softened

Instructions:

1. Line an 8x8-inch baking dish with a large lightly greased parchment paper.
2. In a large bowl, add oats, nuts, chocolate chips, seeds and cinnamon and mix well.
3. Add the maple syrup and stir to combine.
4. Add the almond butter and mix until well combined.
5. Place oat mixture into prepared baking dish evenly and with the back of a spatula, smooth the top surface, by pressing in the bottom.
6. Refrigerate for about 6-8 hours or until set completely.
7. Remove from refrigerator and with a sharp knife, cut into desired sized bars.

Meal Prep Tip:

1. Store these bars in an airtight container, by placing parchment papers between the bars to avoid the sticking.
2. These bars can be stored in the refrigerator for up to 2 weeks.

Nutrition Facts per Serving:

Calories: 265, Fats: 16.3g, Carbs: 24.3g, Fiber: 4.9g, Sugar: 8.5g, Proteins: 7g, Sodium: 8mg

Apple Crisp

Prep time: 15 minutes, Cook time: 20 minutes; Serves 4

Ingredients:

For Filling:

- 2 large Granny Smith apples, peeled, cored and chopped
- 2 tablespoons water
- 2 tablespoons fresh apple juice
- ¼ teaspoon ground cinnamon

For Topping:

- ½ cup quick rolled oats
- ¼ cup unsweetened coconut flakes
- 2 tablespoons pecans, chopped
- ½ teaspoon ground cinnamon
- ¼ cup water

Instructions:

1. Preheat the oven to 300 degrees F. Lightly, grease a baking dish.
2. For filling: in a large bowl, place all the ingredients and gently stir to combine.
3. For topping: in another bowl, add all the ingredients and mix well.
4. Transfer the filing mixture into the prepared baking dish evenly.
5. Spread the topping over filling mixture evenly.
6. Bake for about 20 minutes or until top becomes golden brown.
7. Remove from the oven and place onto a wire rack to cool slightly.
8. Serve warm.

Meal Prep Tip:

1. Remove from the oven and place the crisp onto a wire rack to cool completely.
2. With a double layer of aluminum foil, cover the crisp and freeze for up to 3 months.
3. Before serving, thaw overnight in the refrigerator.
4. Warm in a 350 degrees F oven for about 20-25 minutes or until heated completely.

Nutrition Facts per Serving:

Calories: 231, Fats: 7.8g, Carbs: 38.8g, Fiber: 5.7g, Sugar: 24.5g, Proteins: 3.1g, Sodium: 9mg

Blueberry Crumble

Prep time: 15 minutes, Cook time: 40 minutes; Serves 4

Ingredients:

- ¼ cup coconut flour
- ¼ cup arrowroot flour
- ¾ teaspoon baking soda
- ¼ cup banana, peeled and mashed
- 2 tablespoons coconut oil, melted
- 3 tablespoons filtered water
- ½ tablespoon fresh lemon juice
- 1½ cups fresh blueberries

Instructions:

1. Preheat the oven to 300 degrees F. Lightly, grease an 8x8-inch baking dish.
2. In a large bowl, add all the ingredients except blueberries and mix well.
3. In the bottom of prepared baking dish, place blueberries evenly and top with flour mixture.
4. Bake for about 35-40 minutes or until top becomes golden brown.
5. Serve warm.

Meal Prep Tip:

1. Remove from the oven and place the crumble onto a wire rack to cool completely.
2. With a double layer of aluminum foil, cover the crumble and freeze for up to 3 months.
3. Before serving, thaw overnight in the refrigerator.
4. Warm in a 350 degrees F oven for about 20-25 minutes or until heated completely.

Nutrition Facts per Serving:

Calories: 133, Fats: 7.8g, Carbs: 16.1g, Fiber: 4.7g, Sugar: 6.6g, Proteins: 1.9g, Sodium: 133mg

Chapter 10 Entrée Recipes

Barley Pilaf

Prep time: 15 minutes, Cook time: 1 hour; Serves 4

Ingredients:

- ½ cup pearl barley
- 1¼ cups homemade vegetable broth
- 2 tablespoons vegetable oil, divided
- 2 garlic cloves, minced
- ½ cup onion, chopped
- ½ cup eggplant, sliced thinly
- ½ cup green bell pepper, seeded and chopped
- ½ cup red bell pepper, seeded and chopped
- 2 tablespoons fresh cilantro, chopped
- 2 tablespoons fresh mint leaves, chopped
- 1 tablespoon soy sauce

Instructions:

1. In a pan, add the barley and broth over medium-high heat and bring to a boil.
2. Immediately, reduce the heat to low and simmer, covered for about 45 minutes or until all the liquid is absorbed.
3. In a large skillet, heat 1 tablespoon of oil over high heat and sauté the garlic for about 1 minute.
4. Stir in the cooked barley and cook for about 3 minutes.
5. Remove from the heat and set aside.
6. In another skillet, heat the remaining oil over medium heat and sauté the onion for about 4-5 minutes.
7. Add the eggplant and bell pepper and stir fry for about 3-5 minutes.
8. Stir in the remaining ingredients and cook for about 2-3 minutes.
9. Stir in the barley mixture and cook for about 2-3 minutes.
10. Serve hot.

Meal Prep Tip:

1. Transfer the pilaf into a large bowl and set aside to cool.
2. Divide the pilaf into 4 airtight containers.
3. Cover and refrigerate for up to 5 days
4. Reheat in the microwave before serving.

Nutrition Facts per Serving:

Calories: 176, Fats: 7.2g, Carbs: 25.6g, Fiber: 5.6g, Sugar: 3.3g, Proteins: 3.5g, Sodium: 396mg

Lentil Chili

Prep time: 15 minutes, Cook time: 2 hours 10 minutes; Serves 8

Ingredients:

- 2 teaspoons olive oil
- 1 large onion, chopped
- 3 medium carrot, peeled and chopped
- 4 celery stalks, chopped
- 2 garlic cloves, minced
- 1 jalapeño pepper, seeded and chopped
- ½ tablespoon dried thyme, crushed
- 1 tablespoon chipotle chili powder
- ½ tablespoon cayenne pepper
- 1½ tablespoons ground coriander
- 1½ tablespoons ground cumin
- 1 teaspoon ground turmeric
- Salt ground black pepper, as required
- 2 tablespoons tomato paste
- 1 pound lentils, rinsed
- 8 cups homemade vegetable broth
- 6 cups fresh spinach
- ½ cup fresh cilantro, chopped

Instructions:

1. In a large pan, heat the oil over medium heat and sauté the onion, carrot and celery for about 5 minutes.
2. Add the garlic, jalapeño pepper, thyme and spices and sauté for about 1 minute.
3. Add the tomato paste, lentils and broth and bring to a boil.
4. Reduce the heat to low and simmer for about 2 hours.
5. Stir in the spinach and simmer for about 3-4 minutes.
6. Stir in cilantro and remove from the heat.
7. Serve hot.

Meal Prep Tip:

1. Transfer the chili into a large bowl and set aside to cool.
2. Divide the chili into 8 airtight containers.
3. Cover and refrigerate for 2 days.
4. Reheat in the microwave before serving.

Nutrition Facts per Serving:

Calories: 287, Fats: 3.8g, Carbs: 42.7g, Fiber: 19.8g, Sugar: 4.7g, Proteins: 21.2g, Sodium: 843mg

Beans & Salsa Chili

Prep time: 15 minutes, Cook time: 50 minutes; Serves 6

Ingredients:

- 1 tablespoon canola oil
- 1 large white onion, chopped finely
- 1 green bell pepper, seeded and chopped finely
- 5 garlic cloves, minced
- 1 teaspoon dried oregano, crushed
- 1½ teaspoons red chili powder
- 1 teaspoon ground cumin
- 2 (15-ounce) cans black beans, rinsed and drained
- 4 cups tomatoes, crushed
- ½ cup mild salsa
- 3 cups frozen corn kernels
- 1 cup homemade vegetable broth
- Salt and ground black pepper, as required
- ¼ cup fresh cilantro, chopped

Instructions:

1. In a large pan, heat oil over medium-high heat and sauté the onion and bell pepper for about 5 minutes.
2. Add the garlic, oregano and spices and sauté for about 1 minute.
3. Add the beans, tomatoes, salsa and broth and bring to a boil.
4. Reduce the heat to low and simmer for about 15-20 minutes.
5. Stir in the corn and simmer for about 5-10 minutes.
6. Stir in the salt and black pepper and remove from the heat.
7. Serve hot with the topping of cilantro.

Meal Prep Tip:

1. Transfer the chili into a large bowl and set aside to cool.
2. Divide the chili into 6 airtight containers.
3. Cover and refrigerate for 2 days.
4. Reheat in the microwave before serving.

Nutrition Facts per Serving:

Calories: 269, Fats: 4.6g, Carbs: 48.3g, Fiber: 11.8g, Sugar: 8.8g, Proteins: 12.4g, Sodium: 268mg

3-Beans Chili

Prep time: 15 minutes, Cook time: 1 hour; Serves 6

Ingredients:

- 2 tablespoons olive oil
- 1 green bell pepper, seeded and chopped
- 2 celery stalks, chopped
- 1 scallion, chopped
- 3 garlic cloves, minced
- 1 teaspoon dried oregano, crushed
- 1 tablespoon red chili powder
- 2 teaspoons ground cumin
- 1 teaspoon red pepper flakes, crushed
- 1 teaspoon paprika
- 1 teaspoon ground turmeric
- 1 teaspoon onion powder
- 1 teaspoon garlic powder
- Salt and ground black pepper, as required
- 4½ cups tomatoes, chopped finely
- 4 cups water
- 1 (16-ounce) can kidney beans, rinsed and drained
- 1 (16-ounce) can cannellini beans, rinsed and drained
- 1 (8-ounce) can black beans, rinsed and drained
- 1 jalapeño pepper, seeded and chopped

Instructions:

1. In a large pan, heat the oil over medium heat and cook the bell peppers, celery, scallion and garlic for about 8-10 minutes, stirring frequently.
2. Add the oregano, spices, salt, black pepper, tomatoes and water and bring to a boil.
3. Simmer for about 20 minutes.
4. Stir in the beans and jalapeño pepper and simmer for about 30 minutes.
5. Serve hot.

Meal Prep Tip:

1. Transfer the chili into a large bowl and set aside to cool.
2. Divide the chili into 6 airtight containers.
3. Cover and refrigerate for 2 days.
4. Reheat in the microwave before serving.

Nutrition Facts per Serving:

Calories: 248, Fats: 5.9g, Carbs: 38.1g, Fiber: 17.4g, Sugar: 5.2g, Proteins: 14.3g, Sodium: 100mg

Chili Corn Carne

Prep time: 15 minutes, Cook time: 1 hour 10 minutes; Serves 10

Ingredients:

- 2 tablespoons canola oil
- 2 medium onions, chopped
- 1 large green bell pepper, seeded and chopped
- 5 garlic cloves, minced
- 2 tablespoons ground cumin
- 2 tablespoons ground coriander
- 1 teaspoon ground cinnamon
- 1 tablespoon dried basil, crushed
- 1 tablespoon dried oregano, crushed
- ¼ cup canned tomato puree
- 4¼ cups homemade vegetable broth
- 8 cups canned black beans
- 4 cups tomatoes, chopped
- Salt and ground black pepper, as required
- ½ cup fresh cilantro, chopped

Instructions:

1. In a large pan, heat the oil over medium-high heat and cook the onion for about 8-9 minutes, stirring frequently.
2. Add bell pepper, garlic, spices and herbs sauté for about 1 minute.
3. Add the tomato puree, broth, black beans and tomatoes and bring to a boil.
4. Reduce the heat to low and simmer, covered for about 1 hour.
5. Season with the salt and black pepper and remove from the heat.
6. Serve hot with the garnishing of cilantro.

Meal Prep Tip:

1. Transfer the chili into a large bowl and set aside to cool.
2. Divide the chili into 10 airtight containers.
3. Cover and refrigerate for 2 days.
4. Reheat in the microwave before serving.

Nutrition Facts per Serving:

Calories: 254, Fats: 5.5g, Carbs: 37g, Fiber: 11.6g, Sugar: 34.1g, Proteins: 14.8g, Sodium: 373mg

Pasta & Veggie Casserole

Prep time: 15 minutes, Cook time: 1 hour 10 minutes; Serves 6

Ingredients:

For Sauce:

- 1 cup sunflower seeds, shelled, soaked for 30 minutes, drained and rinsed
- ¼ cup soy sauce
- 1½ cups water
- Pinch of ground black pepper

For Casserole:

- 1 (14-ounce) package whole-wheat fusilli pasta
- 2 tablespoons extra-virgin olive oil
- 3 cups fresh Brussels sprouts, trimmed and quartered
- Salt and ground black pepper, as required
- 1 cup water
- 1 (14-ounce) package frozen spinach, thawed

Instructions:

1. Preheat the oven to 400 degrees F. Grease large baking dish.
2. For sauce: in a blender, add all the ingredients and pulse until smooth.
3. Transfer the sauce into a bowl and set aside.
4. In a pan of the boiling water, add the pasta and cook for about 8-10 minutes.
5. Drain the pasta well and set aside.
6. Meanwhile, in a large skillet, heat the oil over medium heat and cook the Brussels sprouts and black pepper for about 3-4 minutes.
7. Add the water and cook for about 8-10 minutes.
8. Stir in the spinach and cook for about 1 minute.
9. Stir in the sunflower sauce and cook for about 1 minute.
10. Stir in the cooked pasta and remove from the heat.
11. Transfer the pasta mixture into prepared baking dish.
12. Bake for about 35 minutes.
13. Remove from the oven and set aside for about 5 minutes before serving.

Meal Prep Tip:

1. Transfer the pasta mixture into a large bowl and set aside to cool.
2. Divide the mixture into 4 airtight containers.
3. Cover and refrigerate for 2 days.
4. Reheat in the microwave before serving.

Nutrition Facts per Serving:

Calories: 373, Fats: 10.3g, Carbs: 58.4g, Fiber: 6.2g, Sugar: 1.6g, Proteins: 15.1g, Sodium: 696mg

Rice & Veggies Paella

Prep time: 20 minutes, Cook time: 20 minutes; Serves 4

Ingredients:

- 1 cup short-grain brown rice
- Pinch of saffron
- 3 tablespoons warm water
- 6 cups homemade vegetable broth
- 1 tablespoon olive oil
- 1 large yellow onion, chopped
- 1 medium red bell pepper, seeded and sliced
- 1 medium yellow bell pepper, seeded and sliced
- 4 garlic cloves, sliced thinly
- ¾ cup fresh tomatoes, crushed
- 2 tablespoons tomato paste
- ½ tablespoon hot paprika
- 1 cup green beans, trimmed and halved
- 3 artichoke hearts, sliced
- 1 cup cooked chickpeas
- ¼ cup frozen peas
- ¼ cup fresh parsley, chopped
- Salt and ground black pepper, as required

Instructions:

1. In a large pan of the salted boiling water, add the rice and cook for about 20 minutes.
2. Drain the rice and set aside.
3. In a small bowl, mix together the saffron threads and warm water. Set aside.
4. In a small pan, add the broth and bring to a gentle simmer.
5. Reduce the heat to low to keep the broth warm.
6. Meanwhile, in a large cast iron skillet, heat the oil and sauté the onions for about 4-5 minutes.
7. Add the bell peppers and garlic slices and cook for about 7 minutes.
8. Stir in the saffron mixture, tomatoes, tomato paste, paprika, salt and black pepper and cook for about 2-3 minutes.
9. Add the green beans, artichoke, and chickpeas and stir to combine.
10. Stir in the cooked rice and broth and bring to a boil.
11. Simmer for about 20 minutes or until all the liquid is absorbed.
12. Stir in the peas and parsley and cover the pan.
13. Remove from the heat and set aside, covered for about 5-10 minutes before serving.

Meal Prep Tip:

1. Transfer the rice mixture into a large bowl and set aside to cool.
2. Divide the mixture into 4 airtight containers.
3. Cover and refrigerate for 2 days.

Reheat in the microwave before serving.

Nutrition Facts per Serving:

Calories: 425, Fats: 6g, Carbs: 78.4g, Fiber: 15g, Sugar: 11.7g, Proteins: 17.2g, Sodium: 1000mg

Rice & Lentil Casserole

Prep time: 20 minutes, Cook time: 1 hour; Serves 6

Ingredients:

- 2½ cups water, divided
- 1 cup red lentils
- ½ cup wild rice
- 1 teaspoon olive oil
- 1 small onion, chopped
- 3 garlic cloves, minced
- 1/3 cup zucchini, chopped
- 1/3 cup carrot, peeled and chopped
- 1/3 cup celery stalk, chopped
- 1 fresh tomato, chopped
- 8 ounces tomato sauce
- 1 teaspoon ground cumin,
- 1 teaspoon dried oregano, crushed
- 1 teaspoon dried basil, crushed
- Salt and ground black pepper, as required

Instructions:

1. In a pan, add 1 cup of the water and rice over medium-high heat and bring to a boil.
2. Reduce the heat to low and simmer, covered for about 20 minutes.
3. Meanwhile, in another pan, add the remaining water and lentils over medium heat and bring to a boil.
4. Reduce the heat to low and simmer, covered for about 15 minutes.
5. Transfer the cooked rice and lentils into a casserole dish and set aside.
6. Preheat the oven to 350 degrees F.
7. In a large skillet, heat the oil over medium heat and sauté the onion and garlic for about 4-5 minutes.
8. Add the zucchini, carrot, celery, tomato and tomato paste and cook for about 4-5 minutes.
9. Stir in the cumin, herbs, salt and black pepper and remove from the heat.
10. Transfer the vegetable mixture into the casserole dish with rice and lentils and stir to combine.
11. Bake for about 30 minutes.
12. Remove from the heat and set aside for about 5 minutes.
13. Cut into equal sized 6 pieces and serve.

Meal Prep Tip:

1. Remove the casserole from oven and set aside to cool completely.
2. With 1 piece of foil, wrap each casserole piece and refrigerate for about 1-2 days.
3. Reheat in the microwave before serving.

Nutrition Facts per Serving:

Calories: 192, Fats: 1.5g, Carbs: 34.5g, Fiber: 12g, Sugar: 3.9g, Proteins: 11.3g, Sodium: 239mg

Chapter 11 Dressings, Dips & Sauces

Satay Sauce

Prep time: 15 minutes, Serves 8

Ingredients:

- 1 scallion, chopped
- 1 teaspoon fresh ginger, grated
- 2 garlic cloves, chopped
- 2 tablespoons sunflower seeds butter
- ¼ cup water
- 1 teaspoon balsamic vinegar
- 2 teaspoons fresh lemon juice
- 2 teaspoons sesame oil

Instructions:

1. In a high-speed blender, add all the ingredients and pulse until smooth.
2. Set aside for about 20-30 minutes before serving.

Meal Prep Tip:

1. Transfer the sauce into clean jars.
2. Cover each jar with the lid tightly and refrigerate for up to 1 week.

Nutrition Facts per Serving:

Calories: 36, Fats: 3.1g, Carbs: 1.7g, Fiber: 0.1g, Sugar: 0.1g, Proteins: 0.9g, Sodium: 1mg

Mango BBQ Sauce

Prep time: 15 minutes, Cook time: 25 minutes; Serves 16

Ingredients:

- ½ of Habanero pepper
- 1 cup mango, peeled, pitted and chopped
- ½ tablespoon fresh ginger, chopped
- 2 tablespoons garlic, chopped
- ½ cup dates, pitted and chopped roughly
- 1 cup tomato sauce
- ¼ cup apple cider vinegar
- 2 teaspoons curry powder
- Salt and ground black pepper, as required

Instructions:

1. Preheat the broiler of oven to high.
2. Arrange the Habanero pepper half onto a baking sheet, cut side down and broil for about 5-10 minutes.
3. Remove the pepper rom broiler and chop it.
4. In a pan, add pepper and remaining ingredients over medium-high heat and bring to a boil, stirring occasionally.
5. Reduce the heat to medium, and simmer for about 10 minutes, stirring occasionally.
6. Remove from heat and set aside to cool slightly.
7. In a food processor, add the mango mixture and pulse until smooth.
8. Set aside to cool completely before serving.

Meal Prep Tip:

1. Transfer the sauce into clean jars.
2. Cover each jar with the lid tightly and refrigerate for up to 1 month.

Nutrition Facts per Serving:

Calories: 30, Fats: 0.2g, Carbs: 7.3g, Fiber: 1g, Sugar: 5.7g, Proteins: 0.6g, Sodium: 93mg

Hot Sauce

Prep time: 15 minutes, Cook time: 15 minutes; Serves 40

Ingredients:

- 1 tablespoon olive oil
- ½ cup onion, chopped
- 1 cup carrot, peeled and chopped
- 5 garlic cloves, minced
- 6 habanero peppers, stemmed
- 1 tomato, chopped
- 1 tablespoon fresh lemon zest
- ¼ cup fresh lemon juice
- ¼ cup white vinegar
- ¼ cup water
- Salt and ground black pepper, as required

Instructions:

1. In a pan, heat the oil over medium heat and sauté the onion, carrot and garlic for about 10 minutes.
2. Remove from the heat and set aside to cool slightly.
3. In a food processor, add onion mixture and remaining ingredients and pulse until smooth.
4. Return the mixture to pan over medium-low heat and simmer for about 3-5 minutes, stirring occasionally.
5. Remove from the heat and set aside to cool completely before serving.

Meal Prep Tip:

1. Transfer the sauce into clean jars.
2. Cover each jar with the lid tightly and refrigerate for about 4-6 months.

Nutrition Facts per Serving:

Calories: 9, Fats: 0.4g, Carbs: 1.3g, Fiber: 0.3g, Sugar: 0.7g, Proteins: 0.2g, Sodium: 7mg

Enchilada Sauce

Prep time: 20 minutes, Cook time: 2 hours 5 minutes; Serves 25

Ingredients:

- 10 plum tomatoes
- 2 medium carrots, peeled and shredded
- 1 large sweet red pepper, seeded and chopped
- 2 medium onions, chopped
- 1 medium zucchini, shredded
- 7 garlic cloves, minced
- 2 jalapeño peppers, seeded and chopped
- 1 cup fresh cilantro, chopped
- 2 tablespoons red chili powder
- 1 tablespoon paprika
- Salt, as required
- 1 teaspoon dried oregano
- ½ teaspoon dried thyme
- 3 cups water

Instructions:

1. With a sharp knife, cut a shallow "X" on the bottom of each tomato.
2. In a large pan of boiling water, place tomatoes, a few at a time for about 30-60 seconds.
3. With tongs, transfer the tomatoes into a large bowl of ice water.
4. With the tip of a knife, remove the skin of each tomato.
5. In a Dutch oven, add tomatoes and remaining ingredients over high heat and bring to a boil.
6. Reduce the heat and simmer, uncovered for about 1-2 hours or until desired consistency is achieved.
7. Remove from the heat and set aside to cool slightly.
8. In a blender, add sauce mixture in batches and pulse until smooth.
9. Set aside to cool completely before serving.

Meal Prep Tip:

1. Transfer the sauce into clean jars.
2. Cover each jar with the lid tightly and refrigerate for up to 3 days.

Nutrition Facts per Serving:

Calories: 25, Fats: 0.3g, Carbs: 5.5g, Fiber: 1.5g, Sugar: 3.2g, Proteins: 1.1g, Sodium: 56mg

Salsa Verde

Prep time: 15 minutes, Cook time: 40 minutes; Serves 8

Ingredients:

- 2 pounds medium tomatillos, husks removed and halved
- 2 large sweet onions, chopped roughly
- 6 garlic cloves, peeled and halved
- 2 Serrano peppers, seeded and chopped
- ¼ cup olive oil
- 1/3-½ cup water
- ½ cup fresh cilantro, chopped
- 2 tablespoons fresh lime juice
- Pinch of salt

Instructions:

1. Preheat the oven to 425 degrees F.
2. In a large bowl, add the tomatillos, onions, garlic, peppers and oil and toss to coat well.
3. Spread mixture onto 2 large baking sheets evenly and roast for about 35-40 minutes, stirring occasionally.
4. Remove from the oven and set aside to cool slightly.
5. In a food processor, add the tomatillo mixture and enough water and pulse until smooth.
6. Add remaining ingredients and pulse until just combined.
7. Set aside to cool completely before serving.

Meal Prep Tip:

1. Transfer the cooled salsa verde into clean jars.
2. Cover each jar with the lid tightly and refrigerate for up to 1 week.

Nutrition Facts per Serving:

Calories: 110, Fats: 7.5g, Carbs: 11g, Fiber: 3.1g, Sugar: 1.7g, Proteins: 1.7g, Sodium: 23mg

Tofu Mayonnaise

Prep time: 15 minutes, Serves 10

Ingredients:

- ½ pound silken tofu, pressed
- ½ of garlic clove, chopped finely
- 2 tablespoons fresh lemon juice
- 2 tablespoons Dijon mustard
- Freshly ground black pepper, as required
- ½ cup canola oil

Instructions:

1. In a blender, add tofu, garlic, lemon juice, mustard and black pepper and pulse until smooth.
2. While the motor is running, slowly add oil and pulse on low speed until well combined.
3. Serve.

Meal Prep Tip:

1. Transfer the mayonnaise into clean jars.
2. Cover each jar with the lid tightly and refrigerate for up to 1 week.

Nutrition Facts per Serving:

Calories: 114, Fats: 1.7g, Carbs: 0.8g, Fiber: 0.1g, Sugar: 0.4g, Proteins: 1.7g, Sodium: 44mg

Basil Pesto

Prep time: 15 minutes, Serves 8

Ingredients:

- 2 cups tightly packed fresh basil
- ½ cup walnuts
- 2 garlic cloves, chopped roughly
- ½ cup extra-virgin olive oil
- 3 tablespoons nutritional yeast
- 1 tablespoon fresh lemon juice
- Pinch of salt and ground black pepper

Instructions:

1. In a food processor, fitted with the S blade, add the basil, walnuts and garlic and pulse until the mixture is coarsely ground.
2. While the motor is running, slowly add the olive oil and pulse until well combined.
3. Add the nutritional yeast, lemon juice, salt and black pepper and pulse until well combined.
4. Serve immediately.

Meal Prep Tip:

1. Transfer the pesto into clean jars.
2. Cover each jar with the lid tightly and refrigerate for up to 1 week.

Nutrition Facts per Serving:

Calories: 173, Fats: 17.5g, Carbs: 2.9g, Fiber: 1.6g, Sugar: 0.2g, Proteins: 3.9g, Sodium: 23mg

Spinach & Pistachio Pesto

Prep time: 15 minutes, Serves 8

Ingredients:

- 1½ cups fresh spinach, chopped roughly
- ½ cup fresh mint leaves
- 2 garlic cloves
- ½ cup pistachios
- 1 teaspoon fresh lemon juice
- Salt and ground black pepper, as required
- ½ cup extra-virgin olive oil

Instructions:

1. In a food processor, add all ingredients except oil and pulse until smooth.
2. While motor is running, gradually, add oil and pulse until well combined and smooth.
3. Serve immediately.

Meal Prep Tip:

1. Transfer the pesto into clean jars.
2. Cover each jar with the lid tightly and refrigerate for up to 1 week.

Nutrition Facts per Serving:

Calories: 133, Fats: 14.4g, Carbs: 1.9g, Fiber: 0.9g, Sugar: 0.3g, Proteins: 1.2g, Sodium: 46mg

CPSIA information can be obtained
at www.ICGtesting.com
Printed in the USA
LVHW060957100121
676147LV00014B/813

9 781952 832130